Practical social work

Published in conjunction with
the British Association of Social Workers

 BASW
THE BRITISH ASSOCIATION OF SOCIAL WORKERS

Founding editor: Jo Campling

Social Work is a multi-skilled profession, centred on people. Social workers need skills in problem-solving, communication, critical reflection and working with others to be effective in practice.

The British Association of Social Work (www.basw.co.uk) has always been conscious of its role in setting guidelines for practice and in seeking to raise professional standards. The concept of the Practical Social Work series was developed to fulfil a genuine professional need for a carefully planned, coherent, series of texts that would contribute to practitioners' skills, development and professionalism.

Newly relaunched to meet the ever-changing needs of the social work profession, the series has been reviewed and revised with the help of the BASW Editorial Advisory Board:

Peter Beresford
Jim Campbell
Monica Dowling
Brian Littlechild
Mark Lymbery
Fraser Mitchell
Steve Moore

Under their guidance each book marries practice issues with theory and research in a compact and applied format: perfect for students, practitioners and educators.

A comprehensive list of titles available in the series can be found online at: www.palgrave.com/socialwork/basw

Series standing order **ISBN 0–333–80313–2**

You can receive future titles in this series as they are published by placing a standing order. Please contact your bookseller or, in the case of difficulty, contact us at the address below with your name and address, the title of the series and the ISBN quoted above.

Customer Services Department, Macmillan Distribution Ltd, Houndmills, Basingstoke, Hampshire RG21 6XS, England

Practical social work series

New titles

Sarah Banks *Ethics and Values in Social Work* (4th edition)

Veronica Coulshed and Joan Orme *Social Work Practice* (5th edition)

Veronica Coulshed, Audrey Mullender and Margaret McClade *Management in Social Work* (4th edition) Coming soon!

Celia Doyle *Working with Abused Children* (4th edition)

Gordon Jack and Helen Donnellan *Social Work with Children* Coming soon!

Paula Nicolson and Rowan Bayne *Psychology for Social Work Theory and Practice* (4th edition) Coming soon!

Michael Oliver, Bob Sapey and Pamela Thomas *Social Work with Disabled People* (4th edition)

Mo Ray and Judith Philips *Social Work with Older People* (5th edition)

Steven Shardlow and Mark Doel *Practice Learning and Teaching* (2nd edition) Coming soon!

Neil Thompson *Anti-Discriminatory Practice* (5th edition)

For further companion resources visit www.palgrave.com/socialwork/basw

Veronica Coulshed
and
Joan Orme

Social Work Practice

Fifth Edition

palgrave
macmillan

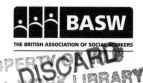

First edition 1988
Reprinted twice
Second edition 1991
Reprinted six times
Third edition 1998
Reprinted eight times
Fourth edition 2006
Reprinted six times
Fifth edition 2012

Published by
PALGRAVE MACMILLAN

Palgrave Macmillan in the UK is an imprint of Macmillan Publishers Limited, registered in England, company number 785998, of Houndmills, Basingstoke, Hampshire RG21 6XS.

Palgrave Macmillan in the US is a division of St Martin's Press LLC, 175 Fifth Avenue, New York, NY 10010.

Palgrave Macmillan is the global academic imprint of the above companies and has companies and representatives throughout the world.

Palgrave® and Macmillan® are registered trademarks in the United States, the United Kingdom, Europe and other countries

ISBN 978–0–230–30074–3

This book is printed on paper suitable for recycling and made from fully managed and sustained forest sources. Logging, pulping and manufacturing processes are expected to conform to the environmental regulations of the country of origin.

A catalogue record for this book is available from the British Library.

A catalog record for this book is available from the Library of Congress.

10   9   8   7   6   5   4   3   2   1
21   20   19   18   17   16   15   14   13   12

Printed in China

To Jo Campling, who is missed by many

Brief Contents

Contents

List of Figures

Acknowledgements

I make no apology for acknowledging yet again the debt I owe to both Jo Campling and Veronica Coulshed for their foresight in recognising the need for an introductory text for social work that goes beyond the basics. Their original vision still underpins the philosophy of the text in that the changes and additions to this edition demonstrate the continuing relevance of theory to social work practice.

I owe a further debt to Catherine Gray at Palgrave Macmillan who had the wisdom to persuade me that a fifth edition was necessary – and the confidence in me to write it. I am also grateful for the quiet persistence of Kate Llewellyn at Palgrave Macmillan who ensured I remained (almost) to schedule and whose thorough feedback, together with that of the anonymous assessors, helped to refine this edition.

As ever the ideas developed in this edition benefited from discussions with colleague academics, practitioners, students and service users. While they contributed much I remain responsible for the idiosyncrasies and any errors in the development of those ideas.

Finally my thanks to Geoff – his unfailing support has been my mainstay.

JOAN ORME

Preface to the fifth edition

Writing the preface for the fifth edition of a book that was first published in 1988 is rewarding but continues to be daunting. The rewards are to do with the fact that the basic idea of the book has withstood the test of time. All credit should go to Veronica Coulshed for that – it was her original idea. However, every time I write a new edition I am daunted by what I see as a balancing act. On the one hand, I do not want to lose the original clarity of Veronica's text. On the other, I do not want this version to be out of touch and therefore not relevant to social work students and practitioners of today – and tomorrow.

The biggest challenge is in the title – *Social Work Practice*. It begs the question 'what is social work?' What is known as social work practice today is very different from social work practice over twenty years ago. Or is it? What is fascinating is how many of the original ideas remain relevant. This is despite political and policy changes that have influenced social work to the extent that even the terminology has changed. Social work is now referred to as a branch of social care. Some, influenced by European traditions, also use the term social pedagogy. In England, social services have been separated into Children's Services and Adult Services. Reference to changing practices in England is a stark reminder that devolution in the UK means that policy determined by the Scottish Government and the Welsh Assembly can lead to different organisation and practices in the different countries.

Over time, social work has changed either in response to policy developments or as a result of practitioners and academics critically reflecting on the role and purpose of social work. There is concern that such changes herald the end of social work. In my view that is unlikely. This text is testimony to the fact that social work has been able to respond to challenges. This response includes the introduction of new methods of intervention, such as solution-focused practice and practitioners working differently within particular methods of intervention, including more partnership with service users. The tasks that social workers perform, the understanding they bring to those tasks and the nature of the relationships they build with people in need remain vital whatever the arrangements for delivering services. I have the confidence to say this because underpinning the changes is a continuing and increasing emphasis on the nature of the relationship with service users. Also the growing body of research and knowledge in social work is testimony to not only the work that social workers do but also their commitment to 'getting it right'.

Debates about 'what is social work?' have been at the heart of international and national debate. The international definition of social work, agreed in 2000 (and currently under review) by the International Federation of Social Workers and the International Association of Schools of Social Work, affirms a shared understanding of social work:

> The social work profession promotes change, problem solving in human relationships and the empowerment and liberation of people to enhance well being.

It recognises that the holistic focus of social work is universal, but the priorities of social work practice will vary from country to country and from time to time depending on cultural, historical and socio-economic conditions. Since the original definition there have been major reviews of social work in the UK. The 21st-Century Review of Social Work in Scotland (Scottish Executive, 2006a) avoids giving definitions of social work, but relies on detailed description and prescription of what social work services should do, and how they should do it. However a discussion document provided for the review (Brand *et al.*, 2005) identifies three main categories where a need for social work intervention may arise. These are:

1. When people know they face obstacles to achieving the outcomes they want to achieve and seek intervention because:
   • they, their families, their support networks or communities cannot overcome them, or
   • the costs (physical, emotional, social and financial) to them are too high in the short, medium or longer term, or
   • the resources needed are so specialised that they are only available through a social work, educational, medical or housing assessment.
2. When people do not seek, or necessarily welcome, intervention because they are not aware of ways of

overcoming the obstacles they face, or lack the information, knowledge and/or skills to do this either partially or completely.
3. The small minority of situations where people seek, or their behaviour creates, outcomes that are contrary to legislation and regulation, or are a serious risk to their wellbeing or that of others, and where compulsory intervention may become necessary.

This can be compared with *The Public Description of Social Work* provided by the Social Work Taskforce (DCSF, 2009) in England:

Social work helps adults and children to be safe so they can cope and take control of their lives again.
Social workers make life better for people in crisis who are struggling to cope, feel alone and cannot sort out their problems unaided.
How social workers do this depends on the circumstances. Usually they work in partnership with the people they are supporting – check out what they need, find what will help them, build their confidence, and open doors to other services. Sometimes, in extreme situations such as where people are at risk of harm or in danger of hurting others, social workers have to take stronger action – and they have the legal powers and duties to do this. (2009, p. 9)

The description recognises that many people do some of these things for themselves but points out that social workers have specialist training, are qualified and know when to use their legal powers and responsibilities.

All of these definitions suggest that at the heart of social work is the need for change. People come to social work agencies, either willingly or reluctantly, because they want something or someone to change for the better. It is this commitment to change that is at the core of this text. However, what is different about social work in the current context is that an acknowledgement of need for change is not defined solely by policy makers. It also recognises what those who use the services want, or need. The public description of social work given by the Social Work Taskforce acknowledges that any one of us might need the services of social work and social care: that citizens can be service users, therefore service users are citizens.

This raises one issue that continues to be problematic in the different editions of this text and that is language. By this I mean language in general but also the use of terms such as 'client' and 'service user' in particular. Over time the shift in terminology has reflected the changing nature of the relationship between social workers and those who require their services. In this edition of the text, both terms are used. Where the original material is retained which references methods that were developed some time ago the term 'client' has been retained. This is because the terminology reflects the theory and values represented by those methods. In the rest of the text 'service user' is used, although Chapter 3 does highlight discussions which suggest that even this terminology is inappropriate.

It is impossible for any one text to cover in detail all that is required for such a demanding, but rewarding, profession as social work. This text is not a 'how to do it' text, a skills manual: it is an introduction, a grounding in the ideas. To this end, it is divided into three parts: social work processes; methods of intervention and contexts of intervention. Social work processes cover the skills and practices that underpin everything that social workers do – assessment, communication, working in partnership and reflection and review. The methods of intervention explore theories that underpin different kinds of intervention available to practitioners – counselling, crisis interventions, problem solving practice and cognitive-behavioural work. The final part – contexts – explores the policies and practices that are pertinent when working with particular user groups. Inevitably there are overlaps between these sections – social work is not a neat profession – but it is intended that the different perspectives give students and practitioners a broad understanding of what social workers do, and why.

It is hoped that the introduction to the theories behind social work interventions and the recommendations and pointers to other sources will encourage and excite students and beginning practitioners to want to learn and discover more.

JOAN ORME

CHAPTER 1

Theory for practice

CHAPTER OVERVIEW
- Why practice needs theory
- What is theory?
- Theories for, of and from practice
- Organisation of theory
- Using theory

Introduction

For social work there is a continuing tension between practice and theory. This tension exists both *within* social work and *about* social work. At times, students and practitioners have protested that it was necessary to forget theory once in practice. The argument has been that theory is abstract, inaccessible, and that it reduces spontaneity in helping people. Using theory implied distance and objectivity which contrasted with feelings and the living reality of social work encounters. As such it was seen to be a stumbling-block to developing individual style, and the most that could be hoped for was that students would admit that they might subconsciously be using theory that they had absorbed during their education and training.

Other discussions that have taken place, mainly among academics, are that social work has suffered because it has been seen to be theory-less or atheoretical. Because social work is about practice it is seen to be merely the appliance of other social sciences (Orme, 2000a). While this might be an academic debate, in more ways than one, it is important because social work's uneasy relationship with theory has made it vulnerable, in many respects. Without a theory base, policy makers could argue that anyone can do social work, or that social work was not necessary. Or they could introduce policies and practices, such as care management, that sought to displace social work to the extent that it was renamed social care. Also debates about qualifying levels for the social work profession have reflected the opinion of some that there is no need for theory and/or research in social work. However for those for whom social work exists, client/service users, the lack of theory can constitute a threat to the quality of services provided.

In a text about social work practice therefore it is vital that we consider the role of theory. This is not because theory should prescribe how social work must be practised. As Ayre and Barrett (2003) argue theory is not deeper and stronger than practice but is intermeshed with it within a reflexive web of influences. Whichever way we look at it, the use of theory is the hallmark of a good practitioner.

Why practice needs theory

Information gathered when working in social situations can be interpreted in many different ways, depending on which theoretical approach is used. It leads to different kinds of knowledge. Early social work approaches, based on a medical model, assumed certainties; that if you are dealing with A, you can intervene with B and that will secure an acceptable outcome C. However it became apparent that using approach B did not always lead to the same outcome – and that approaches D, E and/or Z might be equally effective.

In a developing climate of managerialism this led to negative assumptions about social work: that nothing worked. Workers were scrutinised using performance indicators that included the number of service users or problems dealt with, the time taken to respond to a referral (or to prepare a report) or other calculations of throughput and output. The management 'outcome' was often that the required form has been completed rather than the particular problem relieved. This was exacerbated by the use of technology. Parton (2008) argues that the storage of data in information systems has implications for theory for social work. The need for fast moving accumulation of 'byte' sized databases might negate the need for theories that prioritise the relational nature of social work: those that are 'slow, detached and reflective?' (Parton, 2008, p. 265). He recognises that practitioners have to operate in an 'informational context' but argues for the relational aspects of social work theory.

However this begs the question of 'what works?' or what is thought to be important. The quality of the intervention, what has occurred or might occur between the worker and the service user while the form is being completed or the computer programme completed, was not a priority as reflected by national standards for probation practice, competences for care management or definitions of 'best value'.

The question 'what works?' led to a more productive approach to practice and theory. Managers and policy makers required an evidence base for particular social work interventions. This was however still accompanied by a managerialist approach which wanted to use the evidence base to ensure 'best practice', however this was defined. The search for the 'golden bullet' or the A+B=C formula to interventions was still the Holy Grail.

Theory, practice and research

There is now universal acceptance that a research base for social work is necessary. A number of initiatives focus on ways of encouraging social workers to utilise research findings to inform their practice. These initiatives have been supported by the setting up of the Social Care Institute for Excellence (Scie) in England (and its sister institution the Institute of Research and Innovation in Social Services (IRISS) in Scotland) with a remit to ensure 'knowledge transfer', that is, to gather research findings, evaluate them and disseminate them to the social care workforce. Other examples of support for a research base for social work include Research in Practice for both children and adults based at Dartington.

An evidence-based approach to practice, first described in criminal justice as the 'what works' approach (McGuire, 1995) is now accepted in social work. However the terms 'evidence-based' and 'what works' are contentious (Sheldon and Chilvers, 2001). Debates about the nature of the research, appropriate methodologies, ethical issues and the impact of research are central to social work, both in academia and in practice (Orme and Shemmings, 2010). Parton (2000) suggests that crucial to discussions about an evidence base for social work is an understanding of whether evidence of good practice refers to the way problems can be solved, or the effectiveness of the organisation.

Fears that emphasis on theory curtails the spontaneity and freedom of practitioners are real. But approaches to research that merely describe findings and assume that these are the answer to practice dilemmas are not good research, and do not constitute theory. This does not mean that practitioners can adopt an 'anything goes' approach. In research, as in practice, workers have to be reflexive (Taylor and White, 2000). That is, they do not accept information uncritically and they must be able to test out ideas in the light of practice experience. This has been crucial in the development of good research-informed practice. It has also contributed to approaches to research that involve practitioners and service users in research, acknowledging that the best way to understand situations is to ascertain the views of those in the situation (Orme and Shemmings, 2010). While such approaches are desirable they are not straightforward, not least because they challenge the power of both the practitioner and the researcher (Orme, 2000b).

What is theory?

Educationalists have debated at length competing positions regarding social reality and the production of knowledge, in other words, theory (for discussion see Rojek, 1986; Howe, 1987). Trevithick argues that the difference between theory and what she calls factual and practical knowledge (2005a, p. 2) is that theory goes beyond description, saying how things are, to providing explanations. Put another way, theory provides a framework for understanding a clustering of ideas that attempt to explain reality in a self-conscious way (Stepney and Ford, 2000, p. viii). This self-conscious explanation involves 'making sense' of what is going on by observing, describing, explaining, predicting and intervening (Howe, 2000, p. 81). It is the imperative to explain that distinguishes a theory, which seeks to explain *why*; from a model, which seeks to describe *how* factors interact; or a method which involves formal written accounts of how to do the job (Stepney and Ford, 2000). Teater (2010) suggests that as a hypothesis, a theory is also an idea or prediction about what can or might happen in certain situations given certain circumstances.

However, as has already been stated, accepting a theoretical base for social work does not mean that there is only one explanation or perspective for what is going on or what might happen. Using theory to make sense of situations does help to give some pointers to what might happen, how people might behave and this, in turn, can lead to guidelines on what to do in certain situations but this is not the end of the process. Academics and practitioners with particular theoretical perspectives will observe, describe, explain, predict in different ways and this leads to different recommendations on how to intervene. While for some this lack of certainty might seem unhelpful, Howe suggests that it should be embraced positively: 'Rather than bemoan the number and range of theories the practitioner needs to acknowledge that diversity reflects the subtlety and complexity of the human condition' (Howe, 2000, p. 83).

Also there is no need to assume that, because there are different perspectives, these are necessarily contradictory rather than complementary. The 'gladiatorial paradigm', that is, the notion that social work theories compete and cannot be integrated since they offer opposing interpretations of social reality, ignores the commonalities and interdependence of explanations of how human beings shape, and are shaped by, their internal and external worlds. Moreover it ignores ambiguity, uncertainty and doubt which are features of the complexity of social work practice (Parton, 2000). This unpredictability is also important because it requires practitioners to think about what they are doing, and how what they are doing influences the situation. Outcomes in social work are unpredictable and what we learn from each intervention can help refine theories. This is why practitioner and service user knowledge is vital for the development of theory.

Either/or arguments, such as insisting that counsellors must be either Rogerian or behaviourist, or that social workers are either radical or traditional in their approach, fail to see the underlying continuities that hold together such apparently diverse positions. Most theories have elements in common as well as elements in opposition. The eclectic practitioner, who claims to take the 'best' from different theories, actually holds a consistent view of people and their situations (Howe, 1992; Payne, 1998). Purists might attack this seemingly undisciplined and incoherent way of working; yet this is the way in which practice is generally conducted, not least because it reflects the complexity of situations in which people live and social workers intervene. Such debates highlight the range of theoretical perspectives upon which social work draws, and demonstrate that social work is certainly not atheoretical.

Theory for practice

Since there are competing explanations for the situations social workers meet, it is not surprising that there is little agreement about the nature of theory that is required to intervene in those situations. Siporin (1975), for example, believed that social workers needed foundation knowledge (personality theory, social theory and social policy theory) that would contribute to an understanding of the person in society. Jones (1996) on the other hand criticised social work academics' selectivity in identifying and privileging certain theories or, in his words, 'seeing (theory) as a resource to be plundered and pillaged' (Jones, 1996, p. 203).

As well as different uses of theory there are different understandings of the meaning of theory. Pilalis (1986), for example, studied how students understood theory and identified six 'explanations'.

- Theory as general rules or laws testable against observable evidence.
- Theory as a probability, a hypothesis or a speculative explanation subject to research.
- Theory as a system of principles which help us to understand events more clearly.
- Theory as underlying ideological and value bases of, say, psychological, sociological or political ideas.
- Theory as distinguished from practice ('this is theory rather than practice').
- Theory as idealism and representing unattainable goals ('that is all very well in theory').

In some ways theory is all of these things. A more common way to classify theory is to distinguish between 'levels' of theory.

- *Grand theories* or narratives are those which are now well established and were all inclusive accounts of human behaviour. Examples include Freudian or Marxist explanations of what motivates human nature.
- *Mid-range theories* are not so comprehensive; they address particular phenomena such as loss, attachment, delinquency and so on and try to explain their causes and consequences. Such explanations can be offered within Marxian or Freudian understandings of the world (see Howe, 1987, for examples).
- *Micro theories* describe and explain particular practices such as theories of communication that can be used in all social work interventions.

Healy (2005) classifies theory somewhat differently. She identifies the 'dominant discourses' for social work as being medicine, economics and law. These help describe the world in which social work operates but no one theory is the right one. The theories which underpin social work interventions she describes as 'service discourses'. In describing these, she analyses the different approaches to social work to see whether they are drawing on sociological or psychological (psy) theories.

This group of theories describes theories *for* social work. That is, the relevant social sciences are applied to practice. However practice is more than a 'rational-technical' activity (Parton, 2000; Taylor and White, 2000) of applying knowledge from other disciplines to help social workers decide what to do.

Theories of practice

Few of the grand or underpinning theories for social work include understandings of, for example, what is social work and who is it for. The development of social policy did turn the spotlight on social work and its place in health and welfare provision but not always in a helpful way. For example, criticisms of social work led to policy research which introduced care management and community care, which are seen by some to have led to the demise of social work (Postle, 2001).

Other theories of practice have come from quite stringent critics but have had a more positive influence on social work practice. The radical critique which started in the 1970s with criticisms from both Marxism (Bailey and Brake, 1975) and feminism (see Orme, 2009, for discussion) led to what Healy (2005) has called 'alternative service discourses'. These discourses include changes which involve attention to consumer rights, empowerment, anti-oppressive practice and service user involvement.

Despite a decline in the 1980s, the 'radical kernel' (Ferguson and Woodward, 2009) in social work continues and is sometimes described as 'critical social work' or 'critical practice'. As ever in social work these phrases have a number of uses. For Cree and Myers (2008, pp. 9–10) critical practice is a way of approaching practice drawing on a particular value base that acknowledges structural issues. Practitioners should be part of critical thinking which in turn leads to critical action. For Ferguson and Woodward (2009) the emphasis is more on the recognition of the structural factors, such as poverty, that impinge on the lives of service users and create social problems. They point out that this approach has led to critiques globally of such issues as the effects of managerialism on social work and the treatment of asylum seekers. Their work with practitioners from both statutory and voluntary agencies has led them to conclude that radical social work includes:

- radical practice as retaining a commitment to good practice;
- radical practice as 'guerrilla warfare' and small scale resistance;
- radical practice as working alongside service users and carers;
- radical practice as collective activity and political campaigning.
  (Woodward and Ferguson. 2009, p. 153)

While radical practice incorporates the principles of feminism, ant-racism and anti-oppressive practice and the practice of working with services uses and carers, each of these strands of theorising and practice have also developed in their own right. For example, feminism has not only recognised the potential for oppression of women within social work (Dominelli, 2002a; White, 2006) but has also sought to identify how feminist theory can inform social work practice (Orme, 2001a; 2009). This work has led to feminists, and pro-feminist men, writing how feminist practice also has implications for working with men (Christie, 2001; Scourfield, 2002; Featherstone, 2003; Day *et al.*, 2009).

Developments in radical and/or critical social work have been driven by critiques of how structural factors affect the lives of service users that arise out of political theories, such as Marxism. However, in recent years critiques *of* practice have also been influenced by theoretical discussions associated with postmodernism (Fawcett, 2010). Postmodernism focuses on how and why we seek for explanations or underlying causes, rather than what those causes might be. Hence postmodern notions of practice theories for social work would be 'a kaleidoscope of ideas, research findings, argument, practice wisdom, values and critical speculation, whose coherence would lie in relationships between the different parts, and between them and the reader's experience' (Tuson, 1996, p. 70). These also recognise that service users and carers experience multiple oppressions because they have multiple 'identities'; they can be male or female; white or black; non-disabled or disabled; experience mental health problems and be of all ages (Featherstone and Fawcett, 1995).

The notion of critical reflection (discussed in Chapter 5) has contributed to the synthesis of postmodern critiques and theory building in social work. This synthesis has helped to bring together theory and practice in a way that is meaningful to practitioners but has also led to the development of emancipatory or transformational theory (Payne 1998). As Fook (2002) explains, part of the resistance to theory is that there has been an inexorable link between knowledge and power. Postmodernism questions the supremacy of professional knowledge and thus significantly undermines the professions' claim to dominance (Fook 2002, p. 37).

This might seem ironic in that, so far, this chapter has argued for developing a theory base as part of the recognition of something called 'social work'. But this depends on a particular use of knowledge by professionals. Schon (1987) argues that technical knowledge helps professionals only to a limited extent. Reflecting on the different contributions to any social work interaction involves identifying the limits of existing theories and developing new ones. Hence a reflexive stance requires practitioners to 'reflect in action' and demonstrate or construct accounts of what they have done, in what order and the outcomes; the values, strategies and assumptions that make up 'theories' in action (Schon, 1987). (The difference in the use of the terms reflexive and reflective is discussed further in Chapter 5.) It is this that holds the potential for change (Fook, 2002), not only in professionals' perceptions of the situation that they are dealing with, but also in theories that inform the situation, the theories *for* and *of* practice.

However a truly reflexive stance, a one that develops theory from practice, has to recognise that explanations of what is happening in social work interactions are not the sole prerogative of practitioners. Any understanding has to incorporate the contribution to knowledge from users and carers. Postmodernism questions assumptions about 'legitimate' knowledge. Often legitimacy is granted because of the way things are known, who knows them and how knowledge is conveyed to others (Fook, 2002). In the past, the knowledge, experience and views of service users have been treated as inauthentic or subsidiary. This contributed to the oppression of service users by the processes and practices of social work. Practice informed by user and carer perspectives is emancipatory and reflects the anti-oppressive value base of social work.

The potential of critical reflection is not that it overthrows, or throws out, all other understandings of theory, but that it challenges assumptions that only certain theories are valid. It does not mean that only one form of knowledge, that is either professional knowledge or service user knowledge, is valid; it accepts that both have a contribution to make to understanding situations, and therefore constructing theory about them. This is crucial in the process of undertaking social work assessments, as we shall see in the next chapter.

Theories from practice

Theory that is implicit (Evans, 1976), alternatively called practice theory or practice wisdom, makes assumptions about what social workers do and how they make sense of their experiences. This explains in an organised way how social workers may usefully act, using their knowledge of the social world.

The educationalist/community worker Freire (1972) calls the ability to think and do, 'praxis', a Marxist term that has been explored further by feminist scholarship (Stanley and Wise, 1990). The notion of praxis encourages people to perceive, interpret, criticise and transform the world around them. In social work a lot of time is spent in giving tangible, immediate, practical help, but this does not invalidate attempts to look beyond the obvious to ensure that experiences of inequality and oppression are revealed and challenged. Underpinning praxis is the notion that it is not enough to study the world; the aim is to change it. Hence we have come full circle in exploring the relationship between theory and practice.

England (1986) argues that a social worker's 'practice knowledge' involves a unique understanding of the people who constitute the clients, 'the general processes of perception and the creation of meanings which determine the individual's capacity to cope' (England, 1986, p. 34). However, in espousing a commonsense approach, England is being neither atheoretical nor anti-theoretical, but argues that 'defined' knowledge is not enough on its own. Professional learning has to be accompanied by, or mediated through, 'personal' knowledge that will inform intuitive knowledge and intuitive behaviour (England, 1986, p. 35). This position is reinforced by Parton (2000). His definition of social work as a practical moral activity involves social workers drawing upon tacit knowledge to inform and make sense of their interventions.

Significant in the development of an evidence base for social work is the work of Scie in trying to elucidate this tacit knowledge. By producing practice overviews and practice guides, resource guides, knowledge reviews, reports and positions papers (all available on the Scie website: www.scie.org.uk), Scie promotes good practice by reviewing knowledge to find out what works best and sharing this knowledge with all kinds of people involved in social work.

Other theories contribute to models of how to do social work. Often this theory is developed inductively when researchers or practitioners build up theory from observations of their practice and observation. An example of this is task-centred practice, where a whole new approach to practice was developed after existing practices were observed and new ones introduced and assessed (see Chapter 8). An inductive or constructive approach, that is, building theory from practice and observation is just as, if not more, important as applying theories from elsewhere. As Ayre and Barrett (2003) suggest, the nature of the relationship between theory and practice is not one-dimensional: theory can underpin practice but sometimes it should be the other way round.

In developing a particular approach to practice, a constructive approach, Parton and O'Byrne argue that there has been a failure to articulate and develop concepts and theories for practice. By this they mean 'a range of insights and concepts which had previously been derived from detailed analysis of what goes on between social worker and service user' (2000, p. 7). However, these are, in fact, theories *from* practice. Before considering what that means, we need to recognise that there has also been a development of theories *of* practice.

Knowledge gained from theory exists to inform social workers' understanding, not to dominate it. As England argues, theory is not an end in itself, 'Abstract knowledge in social work, whilst it remains abstract knowledge, is utterly useless' (England, 1986, p. 35). If effective strategies and techniques are recorded and developed, then knowledge is created and can be used to direct others to what is common and regularly occurring in human experience. Some codification of activity enables social workers to evaluate their practice. When social workers evaluate their efforts, be they services to individuals or whole programmes of care, they begin to engage in theory building. Much social work theory derives from someone's experience that has been written down and shared with others. This can be described as theory from practice. However this does not mean that it is unassailable. What it does mean is that everyone's perspective is valuable and, importantly, this recognises the perspectives of users and carers in the development of theory.

But as Stepney and Ford point out, while academics might usefully debate theoretical dilemmas, such as whether truth exists, practitioners can only afford such luxuries if they bring about tangible benefits and lead to positive outcomes (Stepney and Ford, 2000, p. 21). The dilemma for social workers is that there are tasks to be performed and skills to be utilised, but prescriptions of 'the what' and 'the how' cannot be constructed in a vacuum. Social workers, to be truly effective, need to be constantly asking 'why?' It is in this quest for understandings about, for example, why situations arise, why people react in certain ways and why particular interventions might be utilised, that theory informs practice – and practice can inform theory.

Organisation of theory

This chapter has made the distinction between theory that is for, of, and from, practice. But this is only one way of examining the growing body of research and scholarship relating to social work. We have made passing reference to the way that Healy explores social work theory. In trying to put social work theory in context she identifies a number of what she calls 'approaches to knowledge use and development (2005, p. 93). These can be classified as follows:

Ways of using theory	*Service discourses and practice purposes*
Evidence-based practice	Problem solving
Relective practice	Systems theory
Relexive practice	Strengths perspectives
	Anti-oppressive practice
	Postmodern perspectives

This compares with early attempts to classify or codify, which include Payne (1997) who identifies three strands in his analysis of social work theories:

- Reflexive–therapeutic
- Socialist–collective
- Individualist–reformist

While Howe (1987) suggests that underpinning theory is used by social workers in particular approaches depending on the motivation of the practitioners. Hence he identifies:

- *Functionalists*: otherwise known as 'fixers' who want to find solutions to individual problems: to put things right. They are more likely to use psychosocial approaches or behaviourist approaches.
- *Interpretivists*: that is people who are 'seekers after meaning' and who are more likely to use client-centred approaches.

- *Radical humanists*: these are practitioners who feel it important to raise consciousness and are likely to use feminist and radical approaches.
- *Radical structuralists*: revolutionaries or those likely to be involved in the 'guerrilla warfare' described by Ferguson and Woodward (2009).

As we proceed through these lists it is apparent that nearly every-one who writes about social work theory and practice comes up with a new model or a new framework. Trevithick has grappled with this and in analysing the various models has developed ten 'practice choices' (2005a, pp. 81–5) and, in doing this, she brings together both the knowledge base for social work *and* the impor-tance of applying and using that knowledge in practice.

Accepting that there are many influences on the construction of social work theory, and ultimately practice, can be enormously helpful to practitioners. That there is no one timeless, all-embrac-ing theory for social work, and that social work evolves and reforms according to local and cultural conditions of all social life (Howe, 1994) creates the potential to build theory from practice. More importantly, doing so calls into question who defines rele-vant theory, or which theories are privileged at any one time.

Social work theory should never become an end in itself; it can be generative offering new insights and perspectives (Parton, 2000). It therefore has to be both interactive and reflexive, and will change in response to practice constructions (Payne, 1997).

Using theory

Because the discussions so far might seem to lead back to a posi-tion of 'so what?' or 'anything goes', what follows is an attempt to synthesise the many and different approaches that are available to social work practitioners. If reflective practice leads to more and different approaches, then lists soon become redundant. What is needed is some kind of dynamic model to help us understand that good practice does not mean that social workers should be wedded to a particular approach, but that the individual, the person, the service user, must be at the centre of any decision about interven-tion. As Figure 1.1 illustrates all other factors that are taken into consideration by the worker have to relate to the individual in their particular circumstances.

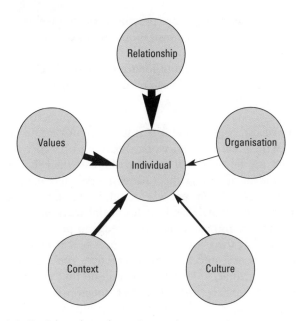

Figure 1.1 Social work as dynamic practice

Having said that, the different 'categories' for consideration have different levels of importance and significance. Hence the emphasis on the relationship: whatever the particular circumstances of the individual, be they violent offender, child abuser, older person with care needs, a young child or a person with severe learning difficulties, the first responsibility of the social worker is to create a *relationship* to try and understand the situation from the perspective of that person 'in their situation'. This is a well-worn mantra in social work but one that is fundamental to social work. The *values* that inform practice include acceptance and respect for persons (Plant, 1973) as well as those that inform anti-oppressive and empowering practice (Clifford and Burke, 2009). But that acceptance, that focus on the individual, does not mean that solutions that are found or methods used, have to focus solely on the individual. Each individual exists in *context*. This context might be their position in a particular family, a particular community (whether geographical, religious or institutional, such as a prison or residential establishment). That context will be influenced by the *culture* of the situation, but culture also includes the political and policy contexts that are operating at any one time. This culture impinges on both service users and practitioners. For service users political ideologies and policies relating to employment, housing, health, welfare benefits, asylum seeking and many other factors will impinge upon their context and their experiences as individuals. For the practitioner the *organisation* is part of their culture. Workers in statutory agencies are bound by particular legislative and policy rules that determine their practice, while those in voluntary and third-sector organisations are influenced by the aims and ideologies of their agency and the resources available.

All of these factors have to be considered by practitioners as part of the reflective practice that informs the processes of social work intervention. This is discussed in more detail in Chapter 5 but the model is presented here to illustrate that the philosophy of this text is not to advocate particular methods or approaches but to ensure that practitioners have a good grounding in the more established social work approaches, can identify what theories underpin them and can make decisions about what approach or combination of approaches is right for this person, in this particular set of circumstances at this particular time – or possibly develop new approaches.

Conclusion

Professional social work practice requires that workers deploy a wide-ranging repertoire of skills, underpinned by a value base that, among other things, respects others. This will enable them to respond to the diversity of experiences and reactions that are encountered when working with fellow human beings. Skills and values are only meaningful if they are informed by theories. However, as we have seen in this chapter, theory building and theory application require a complex interaction between knowledge and process, challenging notions of who produces knowledge, how it is used and what are the implications for practice.

Practice focus

Mrs Jones, a woman in her late 70s, was referred to social services because she was becoming unable to care for herself. The brief referral stated that Mrs Jones lives with her husband and grown-up daughter. Her two sons have lived away from home for some years and visit irregularly.

This case provides the minimum information. In thinking about it reflect on the following questions:

- How might you explain what is going on in this situation?
- What should happen now in this situation?
- As a social worker what could you do in this situation?
- Why would you do this?

When you have answered the questions think about what 'theories' you have been using to make assumptions about the situation. Are there other theories that can be applied? Other ways of looking at the situation? Other ways of intervening?

Putting it into practice

1 Identify a piece of your own practice. This might be a case or just one interview. List all the 'assumptions' that you made when dealing with the situation: about the people involved; what was going on; what might happen; what you might do to help those in the situation and so on.

2 When you have made the list try to organise it into themes around the kind of theory that has informed your thinking. This might be theory about human development, theory about oppression and discrimination or it might be theory associated with a particular way of intervening.

3 You might not always be able to identify specific theories – so ask yourself: 'Where did that idea come from?' and see if that helps you link with any of the ideas in this chapter about the relationship between theory and practice.

4 Finally, think about what you have learned from the situation that you have been reflecting on. Do your particular experiences help you understand more? Do they change the way you think about things? Do they challenge what you have read or learned?

This is the beginning of developing theory from your own practice – so now try to write down the one most important thing you have learned about intervening in this situation. You might then want to go to the Scie website to see if you can find out if anyone else has written about or researched this aspect of practice.

Further resources

Gray, M. and Webb, S.A. (eds) (2009) *Social Work: Theories and Methods.* London: Sage.
An excellent text which covers a range of theories for and of social work. It provides clear explanations of complex theories and how they influence and have been used in practice.

Healy, K. (2005) *Social Work Theories in Context,* Basingstoke. Palgrave Macmillan.

Teater, B. (2010) *An Introduction to Applying Social Work Theories and Methods.* McGraw-Hill: Open University Press.
This text focuses on applying theories in practice.

Trevithick, P. (2005a) 'The knowledge base of social work', in *Social Work Skills: a practice handbook.* Maidenhead: Open University Press.
It explores different ways to think about practice.

Social Care Institute for Excellence (Scie) website: http://www.scie.org.uk/.
Scie provides a rich source of information. It includes knowledge reviews, practice guidance and the electronic library for social care – a gateway to even more resources such as research findings and initiatives such as *Making Research Count; Research in Practice* and *Research in Practice for Adults.*

The Institute for Research and Innovation in the Social Services (IRISS, formerly the Scottish Institute for Excellence in Social Work Education SIESWE) website: www.iriss.org.uk.
IRISS is a Scottish organisation with a mission similar to Scie. Its mission is to promote positive outcomes for the people who use Scotland's social services by enhancing the capacity and capability of the social services workforce to access and make use of knowledge and research for service innovation and improvement.

The Social Work Action Network (SWAN) http://www.socialworkfuture. org/ is a radical, campaigning organisation of social work and social care practitioners, students, service users, carers and academics.
Members are united by concern that social work practice is being undermined by managerialism and marketisation, by the

stigmatisation of service users and by welfare cuts and restrictions. They believe that social work is a valuable activity which can help people address the problems and difficulties in their lives which are rooted in the inequalities and oppressions of the modern world and good social work necessarily involves confronting the structural and public causes of private ills.

PART I

Social Work Processes

This first section covers social work processes. These are actions and/or procedures that are common to all social work interventions and are dealt with at the beginning of the text because they inform *how* social work is practised. They involve skills that underpin all social work practice.

- Assessment
- Advocacy and partnership
- Communication
- Reflection and review

Central to all social work interventions is the process of *assessment*. This occurs at the outset of contact but also has to be a core feature of ongoing contact to ensure that the interventions are appropriate. In recent decades there have been two significant changes in social work driven by different political ideologies. The first is the role of service user and carers in all aspects of social work practice. This has influenced not only the way that assessments are undertaken, but also ways in which social workers intervene. The second, coming from a very different perspective, the marketisation of social work associated with neo-liberal agendas, has introduced changes in social work practice to do with commissioning services and partnerships with other agencies to provide service. These have informed processes to do with *advocacy and partnership*.

Irrespective of what social work process is undertaken or method of intervention chosen, social workers depend on their ability to communicate with service users and carers. A chapter on *communication* is therefore essential in this section of the book which is laying down the foundations for good social work practice.

Finally, as a link between this section and the next one, which looks at specific methods of intervention, the chapter on *reflection and review* identifies the structures, procedures and practices that help to ensure best practice.

CHAPTER 2

Social work processes: assessment

CHAPTER OVERVIEW
- Assessment: theories and models
- Assessment of risk and need
- Assessment and oppression
- Multi-disciplinary assessment

Introduction

The process of assessment is core to social work practice. Increasingly, as the organisation and delivery of social work services change and develop in response to political and economic reforms, the assessment process is the one part of service delivery that depends on the skills, knowledge and values of those who have been educated and trained as social workers. This is not to say that an assessment, or the process of assessment, is unique to social work, but the use that is made of social workers' judgements puts them in significant positions. These judgements are not always made in isolation. The development of multi-professional working requires comprehensive assessment to which a number of workers contribute. However what is vital is that the social work contribution is seen to be an essential part of any assessment.

Assessments, multi-professional or otherwise, take place in a number of contexts and are prepared for a variety of purposes. They occur at the point that a service user first makes contact with an agency, and are used to decide whether services can be offered, what level of service, and who should be involved in offering services. Initial assessments might take place at the point of referral. More comprehensive and specific assessments are required by legislation: for example, those required to safeguard children, court reports that contribute to the sentencing process in criminal justice, or a community care assessment to ascertain levels of need in adult care. However, assessments are also required at other points in service delivery: for example, an assessment should be undertaken when decisions are made to change the intervention, particularly those to withdraw services or terminate contact. Assessments may also be requested by other agencies at any point during a worker's contact with a service user. Formal assessments can be required by, for example, the criminal courts, children's panels in Scotland, mental health tribunals and child protection panels.

Increasing emphasis on assessment has meant greater prescription of what should be considered in an assessment and how this should be recorded. For example, pro formas for assessments have been developed in both community care and childcare, some of which have also been incorporated into computer based information systems (see for example, the Integrated Children's System: cf. Cleaver *et al.*, 2008). Other developments that have influenced the assessment process are policies associated with risk assessment and personalisation.

Assessment theories

Assessment is not a single event; it is an ongoing process in which the service user participates, in order to assist the social worker in understanding people in relation to their environment. Assessment is also a basis for planning what needs to be done to maintain, improve or bring about change in the person, their environment or both. Social work assessments therefore involve making judgements so that decision making can be better informed (Parton and O'Byrne, 2000, p. 134).

There are two major distinctive approaches to assessment – positivist and constructivist.

Positivist assessment

In positivist assessment, a good assessment depends on administrative talent coupled with skills in communication and human relations. This is because it requires an ability to organise, systematise and rationalise information gathered, together with a gift for communication and sensitivity in taking in the uniqueness of each person's situation. In a positivist approach 'hard' knowledge (that is, facts) is paramount; the worker's thoughts and feelings are acknowledged but are secondary. The emphasis in such assessment is on finding causes or reasons for the problem or situation – the worker is expected to be positive about his/her assessment. The judgement making in this approach requires a high level of certainty, and it requires comparison against an assumed norm (for example, of behaviour or attitude). It leads to the production of a profile on someone, the completion of a schedule, pro forma or a report for the court. Because of this, the work undertaken to produce the document is often referred to as 'doing' or 'making' an assessment. Policy guidelines and schedules for assessment are based on a positivist approach.

Early writings on social work assessment were in the in positivist mode assuming there were finite answer to questions (Perlman, 1957). Attempts to understand people and circumstances used to be called 'diagnostic formulations' (Coulshed, 1991) and reflected how early social work drew on a medical model. The assumption was that individual and social problems could be diagnosed and that social work could find a formula or 'magic bullet' that could be prescribed to 'solve' or 'cure' these problems.

Sainsbury (1970) however urged caution in using this 'medical' approach. The inexperienced worker was encouraged to learn the art as well as the science of carrying out this complex task. It was the development of the notion of the 'art' of assessment that led to a constructive approach to assessment (Parton and O'Byrne, 2000).

Constructivist assessment

Constructivism argues that people construct their own social realities (see Berger and Luckman, 1967) and this has implications for how situations are assessed. Social workers making assessments are *interpreting* evidence and should be careful not to offer false certainties, based on particular and partial constructions of the situation: there are no absolute certainties. What is important is how the data on which assumptions are being made has been collected and whose version of events and situations is being privileged. In *constructive* social work (Parton and O'Byrne, 2000) assessment involves constructing an account of a social situation and those involved in it for a particular purpose.

Constructivist approaches encourage workers to recognise that there might be more than one cause, and more than one solution (Pease and Fook, 1999; Milner and O'Byrne, 2002; Fook, 2002). Reflection becomes central to the assessment process. Reflection (discussed in more detail in Chapter 5) in this context involves reconsideration or re-evaluation of the information, thoughts, feelings and understandings that have been amassed during the assessment process. As Milner and O'Byrne observe, assessment often reveals many truths or understandings of situations (Milner and O'Byrne, 2002) but we should not be frozen into inactivity by the complexities and dilemmas that this may create. Critical reflection assists both in sense making and recognising how our own biases and prejudices influence the assessment process (Fook, 2002). The theoretical models that are used to interpret the information are also influential.

Assessment models

The skill in undertaking and recording an assessment lies in the ability to collect enough of the right kind of information. Frequently beginners attempt to find out everything by asking more and more questions, resulting in confusion from information overload. It is as well to remember the following:

- it is not possible to know all there is to know about people or systems;
- assessments are always continuous and dynamic and, in this sense, never complete;
- assessments are never 'true' – they tend to be filtered through the assessor's perspective, despite attempts at exactness and comprehensiveness and careful reflection;
- reflection can provide checks and balances on both the assessor's 'biases' and the possible discriminatory or negative stereotyping that may occur within the process.

Common 'models' of assessment can be classified either by the purpose of the assessment, that is, initial assessment, needs-led assessment, risk assessment, or they can be classified by the way that they are carried out. In the first instance we will look at models of how assessments can be conducted.

Questioning model

The most basic approach to assessment is the questioning model. Dialogue between workers and service users in assessment has to be based on questioning: questions facilitate communication. It is the nature of the questions and the way the answers are utilised that is significant.

The classic questioning model reflects the reductionist approach to assessment (Milner and O'Byrne, 2002). Problems, and solutions, are seen to rest in the individual, and the social work task is to identify the problem and find the appropriate resources or solutions. One limitation of this model is the assumption that there is a truth that can be gleaned by interrogation, along the lines of a police interview. Another is that social workers are seen as the experts who examine each aspect of the system and come to a final decision on the basis of their expertise and the knowledge gained. Such approaches have been deemed to be oppressive and disempowering (Smale *et al.*, 1993).

However the questioning model does not have to be employed in such a negative way. It is not the questioning that is disempowering, but how it is undertaken and what is done with the information. When gathering information it is imperative that:

- hearsay or gossip is not relied on;
- questions are not asked in order to trick people or to 'catch them out';
- open rather than closed questions should be used (see Chapter 4);
- questions are asked in ways that try to help understand what is influencing the particular presentation of the information;
- it is necessary to avoid stereotyping or labelling people as deviant because they do not conform to one individual's perception of 'normality'.

Procedural model

In a procedural model, workers undertake assessment using systems to ensure consistent and comprehensive data collection. Such systems are often typified by a large number of forms to be completed. Procedural models of assessment have been produced either as a result of guidance related to legislation or as a result of research.

Figure 2.1 is an example of a procedural model developed in work with children and families (DoH, 2000c; see Houston, 2002 for a discussion of the development). The model draws on a systemic ecological approach to ensure that the whole situation is understood without attaching blame (Houston, 2002). The background to the framework and the guidance notes provide a wealth of information for beginning social workers. The aim of this

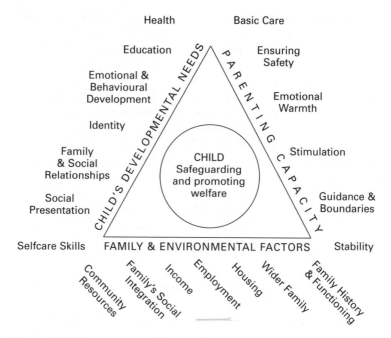

Figure 2.1 The assessment framework
Source: DoH, 2000c, reproduced under the Open Government Licence v1.0.

approach to assessment is to improve practice, by ensuring that there is a consistent approach to identifying need and responding to it.

However critics have warned that, despite the underlying principle, the use of frameworks do not necessarily lead to good assessment. Criticisms include concerns that such an approach to assessment:

- gives little opportunity for the individual or family to 'tell their story': to describe the situation as they experience it;
- constrains the way workers undertake assessments;
- can lead to inappropriate labelling (Garrett, 2003);
- is underpinned by heterosexist assumptions (Charnley and Langley, 2007);
- gives the worker significant power (Houston, 2002).

An alternative approach, which also emphasises information gathering, is found in the Scottish Government's policies on *Getting it Right for Every Child* (Scottish Government, 2008). The use of the 'my world triangle' focuses on the child's or young person's whole world from their perspective and recognises there are connections between the different parts of their world.

The introduction of information technology (IT) systems has influenced procedural models of assessment as, in some areas of practice, data is input into computer programs to facilitate the process of documenting all the information required. This is intended to assist workers collect, share, classify and store *information*. However, such a database culture can have a negative impact on practice (Parton, 2008): good assessments are about more than information.

While there is an obvious need to collect data, it is the use of the data and information that is crucial (Garret 2003). A positive outcome is that data becomes more available and accessible and decisions become more transparent. However there are a number of negative consequences:

- Knowledge, which cannot be squeezed into the required format, disappears or gets lost (Parton, 2008).
- Data is collected for different purposes and can be stored in different places leading to lack of coherence. For example, a financial assessment for community care might indicate that an older person has very few resources, while another pro forma assessing health issues might indicate he/she is depressed because he/she has few social contacts. It is only when the two pieces of information are brought together that it becomes obvious that the older person is not able to go out or join social activities because of his/her lack of resources. There is therefore nowhere for a picture of the whole person to be presented. The emphasis is on *what* happened not why it happened (Parton, 2008).
- Assessment processes that privilege agency agendas, focus on gathering data and marginalise the thoughts of service users, may lead to inappropriate intervention based on inadequate understanding (Richards, 2000). For example, Cleaver and Walker (2004) reported that social workers felt their records were being used as bureaucratic tools to regularise practice rather than respond to need.
- Even with the checks and balances of the Data Protection Act to prevent misuse, information about the individual is collected and stored that does not obviously relate to the problem or issue that has brought him/her to the attention of social services. In both childcare work (Cleaver and Walker, 2004)

and assessments of older people (Richards, 2000), workers tended to resort to questions and answers and focused on the information for the form. Service users can be distressed or angered by having to reveal so much about him or herself that seems irrelevant.

A crucial consideration is service users' and carers' views of assessment. However they can differ. Cleaver and Walker (2004) report that the parents in their study expressed satisfaction with the process of assessment and felt that they had been consulted and involved at all stages. However Richards argues that conducting a wide-ranging enquiry, rather than one driven by schedules, is more likely to enable older people to think through the situation more productively or accept help more easily (Richards, 2000).

Exchange model

The exchange model of assessment (Smale *et al.*, 1993) argues that users and carers, as experts in their own needs, should be empowered by being involved in the assessment. The 'exchange' involves more than merely sharing assessments with users. While emphasising that the worker has expertise in the *process* of problem solving, the model recognises that people in need, and those involved with them, will always know more about their problems. The aim is to involve all the major parties in arriving at a compromise for meeting care needs. The worker manages the process by negotiating to get agreement about who should do what for whom (Smale *et al.*, 1993). The focus is very much on the social situation, rather than the individual, and recognises that people come to social services for help because other support systems may have broken down or are not available. It is therefore argued that everyone in the social network should be involved in the assessment, as each person will have his or her own perception of the problem.

In summary, the main tasks of assessment in the exchange model are to:

- facilitate full participation in the processes of decision making;
- make a 'holistic' assessment of the social situation, and not just of the referred individual;
- help create and maintain the flexible set of human relationships that make up a 'package of care';
- facilitate negotiations within personal networks about conflicts of choices and needs;

- create sufficient trust for full participation and open negotiations to actually take place; and
- change the approach to all these broad tasks as the situation itself changes over time. (Smale *et al.*, 1993, p. 45)

These principles are echoed in the notion of *a self-directed assessment* which is key to the personalisation agenda (see Chapter 11). This simplified assessment is led, as far as possible, by the person in partnership with the professional and focuses on the outcomes that they want to achieve in meeting their eligible needs. The assessment looks at the individual's circumstances and takes account of the needs of carers, family members and others who provide informal support.

The practice of the exchange model is straightforward. To participate effectively people need the opportunity to think through their situation as well as have intelligible information (Richards, 2000; Barnes, 2011). They are not always expert – but they should at least be equal participants in the process of considering relevant information. Effective exchange in the assessment process requires careful attention to what is actually said. It also requires making the necessary adjustments to ensure that those with sensory and other impairments are able to understand and be understood.

Effective assessment might reveal more needs. Giving people the space to talk might well indicate problems that are not necessarily resolvable. For example, when faced with illness (either their own or that of their partner), older people often have to face the inevitability of death. An appropriate response requires not only knowledge of how to conduct an assessment but also understanding of theories of loss and change. It is because of this that assessment should be seen as not only a one-off process but also an intervention in itself, an opportunity for people to articulate their pain and their difficulties. Insensitive and abrupt assessments governed by schedules can unwittingly precipitate this pain but so can assessments which give the service user all the responsibility.

Narrative assessment

Those who support narrative approaches to assessment suggest that exchange is not enough. It denies that workers have professional responsibilities and knowledge that can contribute to understanding. Critical reflection is required to construct a narrative of the '*what*' jointly between the worker and the service user (Fook,

2002). This recognises that workers have some expertise both in thinking about solution development and building solutions with people (Parton and O'Byrne, 2000) – but they are not the only experts in the situation. Service users are not just passive recipients of the assessment: they have responsibility for making decisions and for being involved in the sense-making activities of assessment. This does not mean there will be agreement: 'the emphasis is on mutual exchange, not necessarily mutual agreement' (Fook, 2002, p. 121).

In developing a narrative approach, Parton and O'Byrne (2000) do not totally dismiss the need for questions but use open questions (see Chapter 4) to develop a reflective story rather than a 'cause and effect' analysis. Then, by engaging with the person, negotiating perceptions and acknowledging difference, the worker can 'invite the service user to help the worker see life as they see it' (Parton and O'Byrne, 2000, p. 142). To do this workers engage in conversations which are informed, but not driven, by theory.

Fook suggests inviting the service user to 'tell me about your experiences' can lead to a conversation rather than an interview or an interrogation (Fook, 2002, p. 125). By being involved in the situation social workers can change that situation – the assessment is part of the intervention. Also, by reflecting on situations, the perspectives of both the worker and the service user may change.

In many situations in social work it is ultimately the responsibility of the worker to construct a professional narrative to assist the service user in different contexts: court reports, child protection conferences or case reviews in hospitals or residential settings. In such settings there is pressure to give explanations. It is better to have honest accounts of struggles with judgement and understanding than to search for false certainty (Parton and O'Byrne, 2000, p. 135) but this requires the support and understanding of others involved in decision making.

Assessment as CORE

An overview of the approaches described so far indicates that, at a simple level, assessment is core to social work because it involves CORE skills. These are:

- communication
- observation

- reflection
- evaluation

The skills of communication and observation are basic to all social work interactions (see Chapter 4). However, it is important to highlight that communication and observation skills do not just operate when social workers meet with service users. All information gathering is part of the process of communication. In assessment, workers receive written and verbal information from colleagues and others, which is key to understanding the situation that has to be assessed. Many factors will impinge on a worker's understanding or making sense of situations in which he or she becomes involved.

Observation of the sequence of events is crucial. For example, if an older person is being referred for community care services it is important to note: who is making the referral – is it a family member, a neighbour or someone in the health or care services? What actions have been taken prior to the referral? Does the older person know about the referral? Answers to these questions give important information about the context.

The purpose of communication and observation in assessment is clear. It is to gather information. However, there is sometimes confusion in understandings of evaluation and reflection. Some people use the terms 'assessment' and 'evaluation' interchangeably. There may be an evaluative component to an assessment (for example, measuring if a service user, or a whole care programme, is achieving goals), but in general, assessments are more akin to an exploratory study that forms the basis for decision making and action. It is for this reason that reflection is important. Reflection is a social work process in its own right (see Chapter 5) but also has a specific role in assessment. This involves reviewing the different perspectives accessed during the process of gathering information and being alert to the ways that these perspectives are themselves informed by the role and function of the people involved. Also, reflection requires that these perspectives be reviewed in the light of theory and research evidence.

The notion of evaluation within the CORE skills is an exploration of the effectiveness of the process of assessment, including the contribution that the service user and worker have made. Reflection and evaluation are designed to ensure that the assessment has drawn on as much information as possible (including social work theory and research findings). The evaluation must also be alert to the potential within the assessment process for stereotyping individuals and their problems, unfair discrimination in the allocation of services, and the operation of power in the relationship between workers and service users.

Having dealt with approaches that underpin the assessment process it is important to consider other ways of modelling assessment: assessment for particular purposes. Perhaps the two most important ones are assessment of risk and assessment of need.

Assessment of risk

Social workers constantly deal with risk. Obvious examples are when there are concerns about the safety of children. The assessment here is not just of the potential risk of harm to the children, but also an assessment of the propensity of adults to commit a harmful act. Other situations of immediate risk where complex assessments are required include:

- Mental health assessments in situations where social workers have to make decisions about whether a person should be sectioned on the basis that his or her behaviour constitutes a threat of harm to him or herself or to others.
- Criminal justice social work reports where assessments have to be made about the risk of re-offending.
- Community care assessments of older people where there appears to be neglect and workers have to assess whether such neglect constitutes a danger.

Risk decisions impact on the lives of others. On the one hand people have to be protected, but on the other they should be allowed to live their lives as they choose to exercise self-determination, as long as this does not negatively affect others.

Risk assessment, therefore, involves complex decisions often in uncertain situations – but these decisions require a degree of certainty. What is frightening for social workers in assessing risk is missing something; the consequence of reaching the wrong conclusion; or of making the wrong decision. These concerns are not driven by selfishness or self-protection, although that would not be surprising in the light of the treatment of social workers in the wake of various child abuse enquiries. Social workers take seriously their responsibilities to individuals and to members of the public who might suffer harm or loss as a result of decisions made on social work assessments and recommendations. This sometimes leads to them taking a 'defensive decision' (Kemshall, 2002; Lancaster and Lumb, 2006), which involves a balance between promoting the rights of service users while recognising agency responsibilities, with the emphasis on the latter.

Corby's (1996) categories of risk assessment in child protection provide a helpful framework for considering risk in social work generally. They are:

- preventative risk assessment
- investigative risk assessment
- continuation risk assessment

Preventative risk assessment is often carried out before any intervention takes place, and may influence decisions about whether or not to intervene. It involves making judgements often on the basis of limited information about the potential of harm occurring and how and when to intervene. The most obvious examples are in childcare cases where there is some evidence (bruising, neglect) that a child is being subject to harm. In adult work there are parallel indicators that alert workers to potential harm (for example elder abuse) or in the case of some people with mental health problems, self harm. Workers in some criminal justice cases also have to be mindful of the risks to others and to make regular preventative risk assessment.

Such assessments use indicative factors to inform judgement: to predict. Using the research base for practice can provide knowledge to inform decision making. However, workers need to be able to critically assess research studies (see Orme and Shemmings, 2010). Sometimes results of research are seen to be incontrovertible and used as predictive factors, either to assess the likely cause or outcome, or to dictate the way in which workers intervene. However, sometimes the research is contradictory and therefore confusing (Parton, 1998; Littlechild and Hawley, 2010). For example, in criminal justice social work the development of scales based on research such as OASys to predict re-offending became the norm but the research base was not definitive (Lancaster and Lumb, 2006).

There is also a worry that workers can become dependent on such scales which detracts from practice wisdom, the use of their observational and communication skills and professional autonomy. Good professional practice requires workers to weigh up the implications of research findings in each situation. There must be a mix between actuarial risk assessment and clinical professional judgement (Canton, 2005).

Investigative risk assessment is often an initial assessment into a social situation that has been drawn to the attention of statutory agencies by someone who has expressed concerns. Many agencies have procedural guidelines for how to respond to such concerns. However, as many investigations into the handling of child abuse enquiries highlight, these procedures are not always followed. Even when they are, they do not always help the worker because they are about procedures and not about processes and skills.

Undertaking an investigative risk assessment is also problematic because the worker has to operate in a way which respects the individual, but also gathers enough information on which to base a judgement. Communication processes discussed in Chapter 4 can help, but the fundamental approach is that in these assessments, workers have to keep an open mind: they have to believe the best of people – and the worst of people.

Investigative risk assessment can also have unintended consequences as can be seen in situations that involve domestic violence. Greater awareness of the incidence of domestic violence led to a number of police forces instituting policies and procedures for responding to calls from women who experience domestic abuse. When situations involve children, the police refer cases with an expectation that social workers will investigate the case as a child protection case. This is understandable as there is clear evidence that children are negatively affected by situations of domestic violence (Mullender and Morley, 1994). However a policy of automatically removing the children can imply that the woman is in some way to blame for the violence experienced. The knock-on effect of this may be that women will not report incidences of domestic abuse if they fear their children will be removed. Social workers can respond to such situations under children in need procedures, but a risk assessment is needed of every situation, balancing the needs of the child and the woman.

This illustration highlights that workers have to approach such situations with an open mind, making no assumptions about who might be responsible for what. This is consistent with the social work value of maintaining a non-judgemental attitude: but this does not mean that all judgement is suspended. It is possible to identify someone as being responsible for harm or abuse and still respect him or her as a human being requiring help. The concepts of acceptance and empathy are core to social work. In particular, the notion of empathy as trying to understand the situation from the perspective of another person, while not condoning their actions, is fundamental to trying to understand *why* people are abusive. Only if the causes of abuse are identified will risk assessment be effective, and social workers able to protect vulnerable people.

Continuation risk assessments are those made at regular intervals in situations in which an identifiable risk has been uncovered. These assessments are often about risk reduction rather than risk elimination and are an integral part of the review processes in social work discussed in Chapter 5. Involvement with social work agencies often carries with it stigma, discrimination, disempowerment and disadvantage. Therefore, it is important to continually assess whether there is a need for social work to remain involved in situations.

Balancing the risks of intervention against the risks of non-intervention requires:

- evaluation of the situation in the light of the original concerns;
- acknowledgement that changes have occurred;
- assessment of whether these changes influence the situation for better or worse, or make no difference at all.

Assessment of need

The National Health and Community Care Act (1990) changed the balance of assessments in adult services to being needs-led rather than resource-led. This introduces a level of complexity into the assessment process for workers undertaking them. Need cannot be assessed in a vacuum. Workers often have to assess competing needs, especially those between users and carers. In community care these competing claims were first formalised in the Carers (Services) Recognition Act 1995, which gives carers the right to assessment.

Policy changes associated with personalisation have also influenced assessment of need. A simplified assessment looks at the individual's circumstances and takes account of their situation and the needs of carers, family members and others who provide informal support. As far as possible this is led by the person, in partnership with the professional, focusing on the outcomes that they want to achieve in meeting their eligible needs.

Formalising assessment of need or making policy assertions does not necessarily resolve the dilemmas in practice. If an older woman wants to remain in her own home and to do so requires informal care she might want the right to say who will care for her. The request may be that a relative does the caring rather than purchase care from a stranger. However this might be at odds with the relative's own plans for how they wish to live their lives.

Theories of need

Theoretical discussion of human need helps us to think about the complexity of the social work role but does not always resolve practical dilemmas.

One of the most well known theories of human need is the hierarchy of need identified by Maslow (1954). An individual's physical and emotional needs are identified and ordered to indicate what is the minimum required to respond to individual needs. This hierarchy is often used to make distinctions between what people *want* and what they *need*. Theories and/or political ideologies are used to determine what responsibility government has to meet the latter. Such decisions therefore tend to inform policy making rather than practice in individual cases.

An equally important analysis is that of Bradshaw (1972) who identified a taxonomy of social need (that is a way of organising or classifying need). Bradshaw identified four categories: normative, comparative, felt and expressed. These categories relate both to individuals and to the individual within society. This has implications for policy and practice. Policy for the provision of services is usually based on normative need but situations are experienced differently. Workers have to help people articulate their 'felt' need and try to assess what circumstances are like for each individual. For example, one frail elderly person might feel independent being able to live on their own while another might experience loneliness and fear.

What is also problematic is the relationship between problems experienced by the individual and the responses available, the latter being determined by resources. Eligibility criteria exist for allocating services which are based on balancing resources against need. A need, in social care terms, usually involves a claim for service but, as Doyal (1993) points out, there are no easy resolutions to some of the conflicts around community care needs when there are limited services available. He suggests a 'procedural theory of need' which helps to negotiate what people want, or think they need, and what is available. Thus Doyal argues that 'those participating in policy formulation must include all parties in the dispute' (p. 284) and this will involve users and carers as well as workers from voluntary, statutory and independent sector agencies. The outcome of such procedures is that at the end of the assessment users should know:

- who has taken the decision on eligibility;
- which needs are, or are not, eligible for assistance, and why;
- which needs might be eligible for assistance from other care agencies;
- when, and under what circumstances, they may request re-assessment;
- the means of complaining if dissatisfied.

This means that decision making is transparent. The way information is gathered and the use to which information is put are crucial in ensuring that assessments are empowering and anti-oppressive. This is vital when needs assessments are based not only on an assessment of individual circumstances but also on managerial criteria. Workers sometimes have to explain to service users why a complex assessment agreed in partnership with them cannot be financed. Transparency is vital because front-line workers have to deliver the message and bear the brunt of understandable frustration and even anger from service users who are told they are not eligible for a service. However, if people are involved in the decision making they can usually understand the reasons for the decisions and, however reluctantly, can accept them (Doyal, 1993).

Assessments and oppression

The changes in assessment schedules involving common assessment frameworks for information sharing *and* the facility for self-assessment in policies for personalisation highlight the complexities that are emerging for practitioners when undertaking assessment.

Attention to issues of risk and to allocation of resources is a stark reminder of the power that social workers wield. Legislation legitimises actions taken by workers in the statutory sector to protect others. However, even workers in the non-statutory sector have power from having access to, or knowledge of, resources. Also knowledge of theories may lead workers to interpret behaviour and label individuals. Even when this does not lead to specific actions that might curtail the freedom of the individual (that is by recommending custody for an offender or residential care for a child or an older person), the very fact that someone might be labelled, stereotyped and pigeonholed in the process of assessment is an abuse of power.

The involvement of service users in the process is vital – but leaves front-line workers in a quandary. They have to operate risk assessment and/or needs assessment in the context of limited resources and use solution or strengths-based approaches to facilitate service users to reach a good outcome, without exerting power.

Most policy documents now make explicit reference to the need for assessments to be sensitive and alert to differences in people's background, according to their race, colour or religion. It might be argued that such statements are not necessary. If an assessment is carried out properly, it will focus on the individual in his/her situation, and that situation will include diverse factors including his/her age, gender, race, religion or sexuality. Dialogic approaches, that is those that involve conversations with service users, and narrative approaches give priority to the person's perceptions of his/her own circumstances.

However arguing that assessments have to respond to certain aspects of an individual's identity does not necessarily make them anti-oppressive. Focusing on one aspect of identity, and assuming that this is problematic or leads to negative experiences, can be oppressive and discriminating. For example, assumptions that women are passive, are 'natural carers', lead to assumptions in community care that it will be women who undertake caring roles (Orme, 2001a). It also means that women are often the focus of attention in cases involving children, even when there is a male partner involved (Scourfield and Coffey, 2002). Assumptions of women's passivity or non-violence can also cause workers to fail to identify situations in which elder abuse is taking place. Bruises, wounds and other symptoms might be accepted as the result of falls or clumsiness, and not investigated as possible carer abuse, where the prime carer is a woman.

Gender stereotyping also has an impact on the way that services are provided for gay men and lesbian women and transsexuals. Charnley and Langley (2007) argue that, in nearly all assessment processes, sexual orientation remains invisible or they are based on heterosexist assumptions. In community care, gendered and heterosexist assumptions have implications not only for who does the caring, but also for the services that are made available for men (Orme, 2001a).

In relation to race, Ahmad and Atkins (1996) have provided an important analysis of how racial stereotypes influence the provision of community care services. Other writers on race and social work have highlighted that social workers have tended to view black users who did not fit into assessment schedules as *problems* as opposed to being *different* (Dominelli, 2002b; Bhatti-Sinclair 2011). This evidence leads Keating (2000) to argue that rather than focusing on one aspect of a person's identity it is necessary for workers to understand that there are many systems of domination, which are often inter-related and reflect the way that power operates in society. Over time black perspectives have been important in ensuring that black people were able to claim a space for their views to be heard (Keating, 2000) but there is still scope for improved practice (Newbigging *et al.*, 2010).

In all aspects of diversity, the message is to keep an open mind: do not make any assumptions about an individual until you have begun to relate to them as a person in their own right.

User participation in assessment

As discussed above, one way of ensuring that assessments are non-oppressive and non-discriminatory is to ensure the participation of those who are being assessed. However, this assumes a high level of knowledge by the service user, and implies that the role of the social worker is to facilitate the process of the individual undertaking her/his own assessment. For some service users this is not possible, sometimes their illness or impairment makes it difficult for them to participate, and others are in such a state of distress they want and need support, help and knowledge from people they see as experts. Also, in assessments required by the courts, case reviews and other situations where risks and needs are being balanced, workers may have to get information that service users might not want to give.

It is important to balance all these expectations and demands in ways that acknowledge the role of the worker, but also recognise the rights of the individual. This can be achieved by first not making any stereotypical assumptions about a service user's (lack of) capacity to be fully involved in undertaking an assessment. The Scottish Government for example has highlighted the needs of people with learning disabilities in assessment (Scottish Government, 2006b). If, however, there are limitations, ways have to be found for involving the user in the assessment process that ensure he or she understands the purpose of the assessment, and the reasons why the information is sought. This can help alleviate fears about the possible outcome of the assessment.

User involvement and empowerment are discussed in greater detail in the next chapter, but it is important to remember that assessments are about people and should therefore include them. This is not only good anti-oppressive practice; it will ultimately lead to more effective assessment.

Multi-professional assessment

Producing guidelines that are useful for other professionals challenges the notion of CORE skills for social work assessment. Often the situations to be dealt with involve *communication* between professions as well as within professions. Social services are frequently involved with health services, education services and the police, and are working increasingly with voluntary and private organisations. Multi-agency involvement can mean that service users have to tell their stories on multiple occasions, and they will be heard differently by different professionals. Similarly, *observations* may often differ because the perspective taken by workers within the situation is influenced by their different professional backgrounds and the aims and purpose of the agency in which they work. *Reflection* is often limited because of both the timescale in which actions have to be taken and the lack of narratives about the different aspects of the situation, or the impact of interventions.

Each situation demands complex processes to ensure that the assessment is appropriate, and that the actions taken are effective in the short and long term. This requires information sharing between the workers in the situation. This is not just information about the particular case in which they are involved, but also about agency policy and understandings of research. Communication has to happen at a number of different levels. To assist open communication, there has to be comprehensive recording of information, perspectives and opinions. Crucially in the light of the observations above someone has to take responsibility for ensuring the service user is kept informed about decisions made, resources allocated and dates for, among other things, reviews. *Evaluation* of these processes is crucial.

Systems have been designed to improve information sharing for example the introduction of a *Single shared assessment* (see Chapter 11). However, the fact that various professionals (for instance, health visitors, occupational therapists, physiothera-pists, general practitioners, district nurses and social workers) work together in shared assessment does not mean they will have shared perceptions. As the Laming Report (2003) into the death of Victoria Climbié clearly identified, arrangements for joint assessments sometimes do not work because workers either do not communicate effectively with each other, or they do not always accept or trust the judgement of those not in their own profession.

As Chapter 5, on reflection and review, clarifies the need for communication, transparency and negotiation remain crucial throughout the process of assessment, as does the need to keep the service user, and others involved in the situation, informed and involved.

Conclusion

This chapter has focused on the process of assessment as a CORE task in social work. It is core because it provides an important first contact between service users and helping agencies, it facilitates decisions about intervention, it influences the allocation of resources and it determines whether or not there are potential risks in the situation.

In discussing different theoretical approaches to assessment, the chapter also describes the core skills that are required to undertake effective assessments: communication, observation, reflection and evaluation. While there are many ways of working to improve assessment it is vital to remember that the very act of intervening in someone's life and trying to ascertain information can, on the one hand, bring about change but, on the other, can be seen as oppressive. Even if the core skills are utilised effectively the process of assessment involves the operation of power, therefore, it is important to remember that while assessment is fundamental to social work, social work values have to be fundamental to assess-ment processes.

Point for reflection

Undertaking assessments in social work is an enormous responsibility, but is one of the most fundamental tasks in social work. Now that you have read this chapter:

• Think about the different approaches to assessment described.
• Write down your concerns about each of these approaches.
• Try to identify what these concerns are about: Making a mistake in the assessment? Missing important information? Not following agency procedure?
• Now try and identify what would help you overcome these anxieties: Having supervision? Having access to research? Reading more books on 'how to do it'? Having more practice?

You will probably want all of these things, and others not identified here. There is no easy answer, but it is important that you set up systems that will ensure you get support when you are undertaking this most difficult task.

Putting it into practice

1 When you are in practice you will have access to a number of assessments. These will have been written by different workers for different purposes. They will invariably involve a set of forms. Read two or three of these assessments carefully and write down:

• what information is given;
• what assumptions are made;
• what information, according to you, is missing – what more would you like to know;
• what opinions are given.

Do not do this in a negative way – the focus is not on criticising the writer of the report.

2 When you are next asked to do a practice assessment, once you have filled in the necessary forms, sit in a quiet space and write down the 'narrative': the story of what happened, what was said, how you felt, how you think others felt.

3 Now go back to your pro forma (or computer screen) and compare the accounts. Which account gives you more information? Which gives you a better sense of what is going on? Which best presents the feelings and experiences of the service user?

4 With the benefit of your reflections and the issues discussed in this chapter write down how you would approach undertaking assessments using both the formal assessment schedules (paper or computerised) *and* a more open, dialogic and service-user focused approach to assessment.

Messages from research

Broadhurst, K. *et al.* (2010) 'Performing "Initial Assessment": Identifying the Latent Conditions for Error at the Front-Door of Local Authority Children's Services', *British Journal of Social Work*, 40(2), pp. 352–70. Demonstrates how formalising initial assessment processes (through frameworks and IT systems) rather than improving practice has led to short-cuts and the potential for errors in assessment.

Further resources

Lancaster, E. and Lumb, J. (2006) 'The assessment of risk in the national probation service of England and Wales', *Journal of Social Work*, 6, p. 275.
This article provides an excellent discussion of the different philosophies underpinning risk assessment in social work and gives a critical analysis of risk assessment tools used in social work with offenders.

Milner, J. and O'Byrne, P. (2009) (3rd edn) *Assessment in Social Work*. Basingstoke: Palgrave Macmillan.
This is one of the most comprehensive accounts of assessments in social work, looking at assessment processes in association with different methods of intervention.

Parton, N. and O'Byrne, P. (2000) *Constructive Social Work: towards a new practice*. Basingstoke: Palgrave Macmillan.
Chapter 8, 'Constructive assessment', deals in detail with the theory behind constructive assessment and how this influences the content of assessment.

Scie Guide 18: *Assessment in social work: a guide for learning and teaching;* http://www.scie.org.uk/publications/guides/guide18/index.asp.
This guide synthesises three earlier guides on assessment and presents their findings. It examines aspects of assessment in social work and goes on to consider teaching and learning of assessment.

Barry, M. (2007) *Effective Approaches to Risk Assessment in Social Work: An International Literature Review* Edinburgh: Scottish Government http://www.scotland.gov.uk/Resource/Doc/194419/0052192.pdf.
An excellent overview of the literature on risk assessment in all aspects of social work.

CHAPTER 3

Social work processes: advocacy and partnership

CHAPTER OVERVIEW
- Systems theory as an underpinning approach to social work interventions
- User participation
- Theories of empowerment
- Advocacy and negotiation

Introduction

Although the need to listen to the views of those who were receiving services was first acknowledged in the 1970s (Mayer and Timms, 1970; Sainsbury, 1975), it was not until the 1990s that policy changes developed the language of choice and user involvement (DoH, 1989a). Community care legislation introduced the requirement that social workers acting as care managers negotiate with statutory agencies, third sector organisations and individual users and carers to ensure that individual needs are identified and appropriate services made available. Underpinning this was the need to ensure that individuals are treated with respect and empowered by the social work interventions.

Only minimal changes were brought about by community care policies. Groups of users were consulted and enabled to make demands for services. A more fundamental change to user-led and user-controlled services developed not as an outcome of the market approach to social work but because of a shift in values. Developments in community care occurred at the same time as the rise of the user movement and the formation of citizens' rights groups. The development of a rights-based approach to social work and the recognition of service users as citizens in their own right were influenced more by debates about social inclusion under the New Labour modernisation agenda than by the rhetoric of community care (Ferguson and Woodward, 2009). User-led organisations

(ULOs) such as the disability rights movement not only challenged what they saw as social workers' paternalistic attitudes to those who require services, but also challenged the principles of who provides services. The implications of this required a shift in thinking in social work from an approach that reacted only in terms of providing standardised services for users, to one that recognises that service users should be given the resources to have their own personalised raft of services and that such services might be provided by those who might otherwise be described as 'users'.

While such changes present challenges to professionals who are required by the state to ensure the provision of services, they do not necessarily involve new processes. Care management in community care involves ways of considering individuals within their particular situations which draw upon systems theory (Orme and Glastonbury, 1993). Commissioning services means that practitioners have to recognise that service provision involves systems that go beyond state provision. To access a variety of resources requires both an understanding of the way that different parts of the community interact and skills to operate effectively within them. Practitioners have to utilise skills that include advocacy, negotiation and partnership to facilitate service user empowerment.

Systems theory

Social work has always been required to consider individuals in their environment (Hollis, 1964). However this usually involved little more than awareness of the immediate economic and social situation in which people are situated, and how this impacts on their problems or the way that they perceive themselves and their problems. Systems theory however encourages workers to focus attention on different aspects of the environment. The notion of systems is basic to a number of social work interventions. In work with families, what is happening to one member can have an impact on the whole family and members adjust to cope with it (see Chapter 10). In community development (discussed in Chapter 13) systems theory can be used to underpin work with individuals, groups and organisations. Significantly the Munro review of childcare services (DfE, 2011) used systems theory to identify how the current arrangement of services for children evolved.

The core of systems theory comes from biology and engineering, where the body, engines, and so on, are seen to be either open systems which are influenced by factors outside themselves, or closed systems which are totally self-contained and impervious. Social work's adoption of systems theory views social systems as open systems (Goldstein, 1973; Specht and Vickery, 1977). The significance of this is that:

- all parts of the system are connected, and what happens in one part of the system will have an effect on all other parts of the system;
- the system needs to keep in a steady state (homeostasis) and will always adjust itself or adapt to try to maintain that steady state;
- there is a feedback loop within the system, which provides the capacity for change.

The application of systems theory to social work (Pincus and Minahan, 1973) was further developed by Goldstein (1973) and, in the UK, Specht and Vickery (1977). Working with open systems requires social workers to focus on bringing about change, not necessarily in the individual; other parts of the individual's social system can be the target for change. Pincus and Minahan (1973) identified four systems within social work intervention:

- *Change agent system* – includes social workers, their agency and the policies they work with.
- *Client system* – involves individuals and their networks including family, community and other groups with whom the change agent system might work.
- *Target system* – the part of the system with which the change agent system is working for change.
- *Action system* – people with whom the change agent system works to achieve its aims.

It is possible for the change agent system, the target system and the action system to be the same. In this way, it is not necessarily the individual who is seen as 'the problem'; it might be the way the individual interacts with different parts of his/her system, or the way that the individual is influenced by the social, or other, system. A systems approach therefore allows for an analysis that encourages workers to be more innovative in the way that they approach situations. An example from social work in community care illustrates how the focus on the person and his/her situation, as opposed to just the person, can help reframe the problem and utilise strengths and resources.

Practice focus

Mrs Clark is a 70-year-old widow with limited mobility because she has a long-term chronic condition, arthritis, and has recently suffered a stroke. She has an active network of family and friends who provide meals and company and ensure that she is helped in and out of bed. The bathroom in her council house is upstairs and her increasing inability to climb the stairs means that she is at risk of going into residential accommodation. She is resistant to this and is showing signs of depression – not eating and not wanting to engage with anyone.

The local social services department, in prioritising the community care budget, cannot sanction the expenditure on the work necessary to fit a downstairs toilet. The social worker tries counselling to help Mrs Clark accept residential care. However Mrs Clark's son intervenes and encourages the social worker to lobby her manager. The son also contacts their local councillor. The decision is reversed. After negotiations with the housing department the necessary alterations are made – and Mrs Clark remains in her own home and becomes much more outgoing.

In this situation the focus is on problem solving and change. The work involves identifying the particular system, or part of a system, in relation to which the worker carries out his/her role. In this case, after the son's intervention, it was not Mrs Clark who was seen as the problem but the social services department itself.

In systems theory the phases of planned change involve problem solving over time, and require skills such as interviewing, assessment and counselling. The eight practice skills differentiated for working with systems theory are related to the stages of the work and include:

- assessing problems
- collecting data
- making initial contacts
- negotiating contracts
- forming action systems
- maintaining and coordinating action systems
- exercising influence
- terminating the change effort

The opportunity this gives for different approaches to assessment and intervention does not preclude individual work; in some situations it may be that the assessment concludes that the individual does need some support and/or counselling. Although some have criticised the systems approach as continuing to have a narrow focus on the individual's experience of social problems and ignoring structural causes of disadvantage, it does not have to be so. Jack and Jack (2000) describe the application of systems in what they call ecological social work. Here consideration of macrosystems such as the cultural, political, legal and religious contexts can help understand how structural discrimination (such as ageism and racism) can impact on individuals, the problems they experience and their perception of these problems. They illustrate how systems theory can ensure that an individualised approach is not the only form of intervention considered.

In community care, as the case example above shows, systems theory helps to identify different points within the care system that need to be targeted. For this to be effective, a variety of organisations and agencies need to be engaged to ensure there are a range of resources for care. Personalisation policies have broadened the remit. Service users are given a budget to access their own services from whatever source they choose. Such policies developments have come about as a result of demands for more user participation in all aspects of public provision.

User participation

During the 21st century, the demands for user participation in welfare systems, at both the level of individual interventions and in policy development within agencies, have grown. However, there has been mixed response to such developments. On the positive side, different mandates (user/self advocacy mandate; professional mandates and legal/policy mandates) have brought about change (Braye and Preston-Shoot, 1995). On the negative side, the forces of marketisation, managerialism and consumerism espouse change but in fact limit participation (Ferguson and Woodward, 2009).

The rhetoric of consumerism arises directly out of a market approach to welfare provision which assumes users and carers ('consumers'), on the basis of information given, will make choices about services. There are, however, factors which influence and restrict the choice of services available to users and carers, and structures and processes that deny some people choice (Braye and Preston-Shoot, 1995). Therefore, Ferguson and Woodward (2009) argue that consumerism actually limits choice: consumers can only consume or purchase from services that are offered.

Using the term 'consumerism' in social work not only glosses over the fact that social workers have compulsory powers that limit choice but also denies the power balances within social work relationships. Ferguson and Woodward (2009) argue that, at best, consumerism offers individual empowerment and does not address the social and economic circumstances and structural inequalities which contribute to, and sometimes cause, social problems.

Effective user participation requires frontline workers to 'go the extra mile' (Ferguson and Woodward, 2009, p. 117). Many do, but more often than not they have the responsibility without there being extra resources to support the necessary changes in practice. To bring about systemic change in user involvement/ participation social work organisations have to be challenged. The fact that an agency has a value base that espouses user involvement will not guarantee that users will be involved in decision making. For example, in one organisation that tried to implement direct payments there were many barriers both at the level of individual workers and the organisation (Ellis, 2007). Lack of policy awareness and paternalistic attitudes, based on concerns about risk and user control of budgets, are often fostered by agencies that do not provide proper training and hold individual workers to account.

This highlights that practices need to be carefully considered to ensure that they are truly empowering. For example, user consultation is complex and does not necessarily constitute full user participation. Methods have be used to access the greatest number of users. Principles for involving users in consultation include:

- ensure all communication is jargon free;
- access a truly representative sample of users;
- be clear to users how their views will be put into effect.

All of these are at one level very simple but, depending on the context and culture of organisations, it may be very difficult to adhere to them.

Significantly, in the 'bigger' picture of primary care trusts and voluntary organisations there is growing evidence of user consultation and involvement. It is becoming the norm in voluntary mental health projects for service users to sit on interviewing committees for staff appointments. Also primary care trusts in health have service users both attending and addressing their meetings. However, there are dangers that this is window dressing and/or tokenism. Consultation should involve full participation in decisions about the way services are to be offered. This might include the range of services available, policies on eligibility criteria and charging for services, and policies that will impact directly upon how services are delivered. When they are consulted at this level users feel fully involved. While this requires changes in organisational procedures, it also requires each individual worker to uphold the principles of empowerment, otherwise the procedures become patronising rather than participatory (Orme, 2000b).

Practice focus

The 21st Review of Social Work in Scotland (Scottish Executive, 2006a) was set up to 'make best use of valuable social work resources and to strengthen the contribution of social work to the delivery of integrated services' (Scottish Executive, 2006a). Service user and carer organisations had representatives on the main panel but, in addition, a Service User and Carer Panel was established which worked alongside the main panel and reported directly to it (as did panels of practitioners and other stakeholders). The panel was supported by the Scottish Consortium for Learning Disability.

The Service User and Carer Panel sought the views of service users across Scotland and was involved in all consultation processes. It also held a series of citizens' juries. This involved a panel (or jury) of service users and carers inviting leaders of different aspects of social work (e.g. politicians, civil servants, Directors of Social Services, Heads of Social Work Courses) to attend a 'hearing'. The panel put a series of questions to those invited to attend. There were both general questions about how service users and carers were involved in the organisation the individual represented – and specific challenges to each organisation. The results of these jury deliberations contributed to the Report of the Service Users Group which fed into the final report (Scottish Executive, 2006a). The final report also carried a specific introduction for service users and carers and was available in multi-formats.

The *Implementation Plan* (Scottish Executive, 2006a) established a User and Carer Forum to provide an opportunity 'for users and carers to directly influence and shape the detail of implementation at national level' (p. 3) and provide specific expertise to ensure service users' and carers' voices are heard within change networks. The Scottish Consortium for Learning Disability has responsibility for managing and facilitating the forum and ensuring that 'hard to reach' groups such as children and the users of criminal justice services are considered (Scottish Executive, 2006a, p. 3). The aim is to enshrine the role of service users and carers in the design and delivery of services through the development of citizens' leadership programmes.

Challenges to user participation

Despite the good example set by the Scottish Executive, challenges to such levels of participation remain. These include:

1. Statutory agencies are not practised in open decision making with the consumers of their services, and because of this workers are not used to asking the opinions of the users.
2. There are situations where users themselves do not expect to be involved in decision making – and indeed might not want to be.
3. There is sometimes an expectation that professionals should know the answers.
4. There are users who have not normally been consulted or involved, despite the fact that they would wish to be. One explanation of this is that some groups, such as children, asylum seekers and refugees and those who require different communication methods, are said to be 'hard to reach'.
5. There are debates about the appropriateness of defining those who come to services 'involuntarily' as users, such as those subject to criminal justice social work supervision.

These challenges are important and have implications for inclusive participation and rights-based approaches in social work (Ferguson and Woodward, 2009). They also raise questions of terminology. As is pointed out in the Introduction the use of the word 'client' which was prevalent in the first edition of this text is no longer acceptable and the more frequently used term is 'service user'. However the *Changing Lives Implementation Plan* (Scottish Executive, 2006a) states that users should be seen as having *expertise*. The term 'experts by experience' has been used increasingly to acknowledge that service users have a specialist knowledge base rooted in the individual's experience of using services (McLaughlin, 2009). All terminology is problematic because the words we use identify power dimensions. McLaughlin's suggestion that terms such as 'experts by experience' are descriptive not of a person, but of a relationship (McLaughlin, 2009, p. 1114), is useful as it helps clarify that users, by virtue of experiencing some difficulties, are not necessarily expert in all social work but they are the experts in their particular situation. It is likely that debates will continue and new terminology introduced but what is vital is that practitioners are aware of the implications of the terminology they use.

Reluctance or resistance on behalf of workers to user involvement arises not necessarily because they do not support the need for change but because such change might be time-consuming, and they have no spare capacity to respond to the extra demands. This is especially so in systems which are becoming more managerial (Ferguson and Woodward, 2009). Also user involvement and participation require resources. At a minimum, payments for users' and carers' expenses to attend meetings are required, but other payments might also be necessary – it should not be assumed that service users, or those representing them, are sitting at home waiting to be consulted. Compensation for lost earnings or payment for attendance sometimes makes demands on an already stretched budget. To be effective requires that users and carers are offered training if they are to operate at the level of expert – but this involves even more time and commitment from all concerned.

Finally, arguments for user participation are invariably couched as user-and-carer involvement. However this suggests that users and carers are a homogeneous group, and ignores the possibility that there may be conflict of interests, for example, between users and carers, between different user groups and even within user groups. Differences within user groups, based on, for example, age, gender, level of (dis)ability, race, sexuality, have to be recognised and worked with positively, not seen as problems.

Practice implications

Practice guidance and research literature have explored the implications for practitioners of user participation and have identified a continuum from individual focus to organisational focus that includes:

- involvement in needs-led assessments;
- consultation about care plans (for example, care planning approach in mental health, family group conferences in child and family work);
- involvement in care provision;

- direct payments (Community Care (Direct Payments) Act 1996);
- personalisation;
- advocacy;
- commissioning services from user-led organisations;
- user involvement in policy and planning.

These different approaches indicate that user participation operates at a number of levels:

- *individual* – how individuals are involved in having their needs met (for example assessments, contract work, strengths based approaches);
- *organisational* – agencies set up systems for groups of users (for example consultation forum, questionnaires);
- *groups* – how user groups influence policy; undertake advocacy; provide their own organisations.

At an individual level, strategies for involving users include:

- encouraging users to describe their own needs through the construction of jointly constructed problems, goals and tasks;
- involving users in their assessment and sharing it with the user (including the written assessment), explaining why particular services are being offered and giving users the right to refuse what is being offered;
- ensuring that users have sufficient information both about the decisions made, and the services available. This is increasingly done through person centred planning (see Chapter 13).

Work in this area has had a long history. The Social Work in Partnership (SWIP) project was one of the earliest (Marsh and Fisher, 1992; Coulshed and Orme, 2006). Such projects reflect the value base of social work and involve empowerment (Braye and Preston-Shoot, 1995), participation and citizenship. The concept of citizenship brings more radical approaches to models of user involvement and participation. These recognise the collective action of people who are usually defined by social care categories (Beresford, 2000), and require that social workers engage with, and commission services from, user-led and user-controlled organisations. While this is a position to be supported, it is not always straightforward, as a number of research projects have demonstrated (see Kemshall and Littlechild, 2000; Robson *et al.*, 2003).

Empowerment

Discussions about user involvement repeatedly draw on notions of empowerment. While the principles of empowerment are frequently invoked in all aspects of social work practice, it is one that is extremely complex to put into practice.

One way of empowering users is to give them the means to exit services or to give them a voice (Means *et al.*, 2003). 'Voice' is exercised by or on behalf of those who want to remain, or have no choice about remaining, within community care services. Voice mechanisms are particularly important for potential users who need to influence services right from the outset, before becoming part of them, for example, to ensure that they get access to a full assessment.

Exit mechanisms are relevant to those already in the system. To express dissatisfaction by leaving, you have to be in receipt of the service. You also have to have the means to exit. This is why, for some, the economic power of having the capacity to control how care is provided and by whom, is the ultimate power. The introduction of direct payments and personalised budgets might be the ultimate 'exit' strategy. They provide the financial means to certain groups to arrange their own services, and, just as importantly, the power to influence the range of services available. This affords them status as active citizens through having choices about involvement, not just that of a passive consumer who chooses from a limited range of available services. However, for a variety of reasons purchasing power is not available to all users of community care services, nor is it attractive to or appropriate for all user groups (Barnes, 2011).

For some (for example, those who are detained under mental health legislation or those receiving criminal justice social work supervision) exit is not an option, but they still have a right to be heard, to have a voice. This is controversial and debates about whether prisoners should have a vote highlight the level of feeling that is generated by such a suggestion.

Empowering users by voice involves conferring rights, an approach that has been at the centre of the campaign of the disability movement, and is often linked to discussions about citizenship. Citizenship entails being able to participate in society and fulfil one's own potential. As Coote argues, 'it follows that each individual citizen should be equally able (or "empowered") to do so' (Coote, 1992, p. 4). Becoming a 'user' of social work services should not deny people their rights as citizens.

Social work literature on empowerment resists giving simplistic definitions of empowerment but concentrates on the processes. Adams (1996, pp. 12–15) gives some useful observations on some of the risks associated with empowering practice or practising empowerment:

- The practice of empowering should not involve doing people's empowering for them.
- One person's empowerment might be another person's disempowerment.
- Be aware of the danger of dilution – from empowerment to enablement.
- Be aware of the danger of addressing too many target groups and addressing none adequately.
- There is an ambiguous relationship between self-help and empowerment.

In social work, empowerment sometimes operates because workers have power *over* service users and this is hard to relinquish (Dominelli, 2000). If empowerment is seen to operate at the level of the individual then power is assumed to pass from one person to another in interpersonal relations: the social worker 'gives' power to the service user. If it is seen to operate at the structural level, empowerment involves the transfer of power across social categories: service users 'gain' power. But both of these models treat power as a commodity, as some concrete and finite substance that can be passed around, quantified or apportioned: the worker acts to empower the user; the user becomes more powerful.

Alternatively power is assumed to be situated in external structures and in ways of thinking which can be challenged. However even such challenges can involve the 'disempowering experience of empowerment' (Fook, 2002, p. 51). For example, if empowerment is about giving power to the powerless, who defines who is powerless? Often attributing labels and categories to people is potentially dehumanising and discriminating. This can be particularly so in social work, where categories for community care make stereotypical assumptions about the groups who require services (e.g. older people, people with disabilities, people with mental health problems) and deny them their individual identity (Orme, 2001a). Equally disempowering is the assumption that certain groups are disadvantaged: 'In the very act of defining disadvantage in order to empower we in fact create disadvantage and disempower' (Fook, 2002, p. 51).

Empowering practice does not mean specific ways of intervening but involves ways of thinking about all situations in which social workers are practising. This requires that workers:

- analyse and reflect on situations;
- redefine and reconceptualise power relations and structures through dialogue and communication;
- negotiate a changed system of power relations and structures; and
- reconstruct and reconceptualise the situation in ways that are empowering for all parties. (Fook, 2002)

Such frameworks provide excellent guides to the way that we must approach practice at the level of individual interventions. They seek to ensure that users and carers are viewed as partners, whether we are assessing someone for a package of care, or providing a service in a care plan that has been devised.

Advocacy

If we return to the case of Mrs Clark above, we can see that sometimes it is not the service user who is directly empowered but that others, relatives and/or carers, have to exercise power on their behalf by using advocacy. In systems terms this can be advocacy with the individual social worker, the team manger, the whole organisation or even with political bodies (local and national) who develop policies. However, it should not automatically be assumed that relatives and/or friends could or should act as an advocate. Often people come to the attention of statutory services because they are without friends or relations, or are currently not in contact with them. Where a relative or friend is available he or she might not always be independent; he/she may be involved in the caring and support in some way and therefore might have a vested interest in the outcomes of decisions.

Advocacy, especially self-advocacy, is user-led and arises directly out of recognition that services have traditionally disempowered users. Like participation, it depends upon understandings of citizenship that recognise the rights of all to participate in definitions of need and decisions about how those needs may be met. This does not assume that all needs will be met, but that the processes of decision making will be transparent and informed by the views of those who have the experience of operating as active agents within the system (Doyal and Gough, 1991).

Advocacy shares many of the principles and values of social work (Ferguson and Woodward, 2009). However, advocacy can prove challenging to practitioners because of the tension between care and control inherent in the social work role. In addition, the processes of advocacy are complicated when the social worker might be seen to be acting for one party against the other, even though they have some responsibility to all: as may occur in childcare cases. It is therefore useful to look at different forms of advocacy.

Types of advocacy

At the organisational level, children's rights enshrined in legislation have led to arrangements for children's advocacy. The office of Children's Commissioner has different powers in the four different countries of the UK but, generally, has been created to generate widespread awareness and understanding of the rights of children and young people and consider and review the adequacy and effectiveness of any law, policy and practice as it relates to the rights of children and young people. In England, a parallel but less powerful role is that of the 'czar' for older people who advocates at the policy level.

The most well-established form of advocacy is legal representation, where expertise, knowledge and experience combine to ensure that arguments are put in such a way as to present an individual appropriately to the particular system, be it court, tribunal or organisation.

Other forms of advocacy include the notion of befriending (this involves being with a person to offer support, rather than act on his/her behalf) and representation. In most aspects of social work the role of independent organisations to lobby the agency or provide advocacy services has grown. Organisations such as *Barnardo's* and *Who Cares? Scotland* have pioneered rights-based approaches to working with children. They have provided advocacy but more importantly, have enabled children to become advocates in their own right.

Advocacy needs differ between user groups. For certain user groups, for example those with mental health problems, their situation might require intense periods of advocacy combined with an assurance that the service is available at short notice. There will be times, of course, when they are able to act as self-advocates. Older people and people with disabilities may have more sporadic contact with independent advocacy services, and may be more ready to advocate on their own behalf. There has been a growing increase in the number of self-advocacy groups in the field of learning disabilities (Lawton, 2007).

Independent advocates (*citizen advocacy*) work on a one-to-one basis. Volunteers act on behalf of those who require services, representing their views where needed. This form of lay advocacy, developed to promote the rights, interests and acceptance of people with learning disabilities, has now been extended to other groups. It specifically recognises that long-term service users are sometimes unable, or are denied the means, to have a voice and that this leads to powerlessness and devaluation. Basic to citizen advocacy is the belief that all people have value and rights, and its objective is to empower those who have been kept powerless and/or excluded by empowering people (including the excluded), and enabling them to obtain the rights of citizenship.

The one-to-one relationship is important, as is the understanding that the person with the disability has been devalued, but it means that the citizen advocate works at an individual level in terms of both the advocacy relationship, and the relationship of the user/carer to the service delivery organisations.

Self-advocacy involves training and group support to help people learn skills and gain emotional strength to advocate for her/himself. It is about personal and political needs, about being involved in a range of activities, and utilising skills that ensure participation. The self-advocacy movement is associated with a reformist approach focusing on participation in all areas of service planning and delivery, as well as responding to the needs of individuals at any one time. The aim therefore is not just to improve services but also to improve the status of service users.

As well as making it easier for individuals to be assertive, self-advocacy has the important function of facilitating collective action. Sometimes professionals display 'benign paternalism' towards users and carers. For self-advocacy to be effective professionals need to be prepared to recognise the advocates and ensure not only that advocates have a voice, but also that they have access to the necessary information and training to make that voice effective.

Lawton (2007), working with people with learning disabilities, summarises what has been written about self-advocacy:

- Self-advocacy should make a difference – not just in learning disability services, but in all areas of people's lives.

- People with a learning disability are interested in lots of different things and don't just want to talk about learning disability issues.
- People with a learning disability want support to see the links between issues in their own lives and other people or organisations such as community groups, political parties and parent groups.
- Involvement should be genuine, not just 'tick a box'.
- Real honesty is needed about what people can or cannot change.
- People with a learning disability want a chance to talk about the things that are important to them – not agendas set by other people.
- It is important to find out what organisations (e.g. partnership boards) think – what problems they face and what they need to know to involve people better. (Lawton, 2007, pp. 43–4)

Group advocacy brings together people with similar interests, so that they operate as a group to represent their shared interests. Groups can include users, carers and professionals, and advocacy is usually at the level of collective or organisation, rather than at the individual level. However, the aim is to be involved in service delivery decisions, to reframe how certain problems or groups of users are perceived, and to ensure that users and carers are involved in the decision making, shared with other forms of advocacy. Group advocacy may well be subsumed under the umbrella of campaigning organisations operating in the voluntary sector and there are excellent examples of the political campaigns that have been influential in Scottish policy making (Ferguson and Woodward, 2009).

Support for advocacy

In addition to being equipped with skills for acting as advocates themselves (Dalrymple and Burke, 1995), social workers are increasingly expected to work in ways that put users in touch with independent advocates and to be able to work with those who are advocating on behalf of users and carers. Skills involved include:

- ensuring all involved have access to necessary information;
- being available to meet with the advocate;
- giving advocates a role in relation to the decision making;

- acknowledging that different user/advocate relationships will have different balances of involvement liaison and consultation, but recognise confidentiality, and respect the user.

Professionals can support advocacy projects, making skills available and accessing resources and information, but some argue that it is difficult for professionals to avoid bureaucratic and managerialist pressures, which limit the amount of power they can give to the advocate. The real test of effectiveness is the extent to which advocacy movements can challenge the power of professionals. Furthermore, the response of professionals to individual users who are advocating on their own behalf requires a shift of emphasis in the relationship, recognising the power imbalances that have traditionally existed within social work practice. Much of this requires negotiation.

Negotiating

The above discussions highlight that in addition to one-to-one work with service users, social work increasingly involves negotiation: with advocates, other professionals, representatives of voluntary and private organisations as service provides.

Payne (1986) suggested the purpose of negotiation is to influence in order to get a just outcome. Negotiation can therefore be both competitive and collaborative (Payne, 1986). Where the social worker has to fight to secure justice or combat the abuse of power, perhaps by a higher authority, then competitive tactics are in order. Where parties are negotiating towards agreement rather than to gain advantage, then collaborative elements are to the fore. Trevithick's (2005a) view is that negotiation is primarily about reaching some form of agreement or understanding and one way to achieve this is to explore the perceptions of those involved by entering into a dialogue and facilitating effective communication.

In social work practice, drawing on systems theory, much negotiation is about working with different parts of a wider system. This might involve:

- stimulating voluntary sector community care services;
- persuading other statutory agencies to honour their reposnibilities;
- negotiating residential accommodation or family care;
- persuading schools to cope with disruptive pupils;

- constructing appropriate community sentences for offenders;
- inducing policy-makers to fund new projects or helping to resolve staff disputes in day and residential centres;
- welfare rights work.

Many of the communication skills identified in the next chapter can contribute to becoming a skilled negotiator.

Practice focus

Paula (a single parent) was referred to children's services anonymously by her neighbours, who complained that her two children were at risk: being brought up in a house that was used by drug addicts, 'dossers' and other 'down-and-outs'. Before the social worker could visit, the police became involved and insisted that the children be taken from their mother. A social work visit established that Paula did have others staying with her. They exploited her limited intelligence, refusing to move out until forced to do so by the police. In the meantime, her home had been wrecked by, among other things, savage dogs. The crisis was so severe that, coupled with her lack of social skills, Paula was quite unable to discuss her situation with the social worker.

The social worker negotiated with police offers at the house to let her help Paula without resorting to the need to receive the children into care. The police and the housing department were identified as part of Paula's system where social work intervention in the form of negotiation and advocacy was necessary. The police were persuaded to help to deal with the dogs. Paula and her children were accommodated in a homeless families' unit to stay while the social worker negotiated alternative housing with the housing department.

This goal of rehousing demanded the most careful preparation, especially as Paula lived in the district's worst quarter, where the poorest tenants were housed until they 'proved' to the housing department that they were 'fit enough people' to be transferred into less temporary property. The social worker resisted attacking council policy or challenging the attitudes of housing personnel. She presented a clear, well thought-through plan for preventing Paula and her children needing to be kept in the homeless unit. The offer of another house, though not much of an improvement on the former, was a start.

The social worker had to advocate to her own department and other agencies in the system to address their concerns about Paula's capacity for 'good enough' parenting.

Conclusion

This chapter has illustrated that increasingly social workers have to review the way that they work with service users – both individuals and groups. Policy initiatives have included lip service to consultation with users, but the user movement has been far more influential in requiring social workers to reflect on the nature of their relationships. Notions of user involvement are underpinned by understandings of how power operates in relationships especially when social workers have responsibility to provide services, protect users and balance competing needs. All aspects of user involvement require the principles of partnership.

Other changes in the delivery of social work based on policies and ideology mean that there is an ever changing relationship between practitioners and others – whether that be service users, carers, other professionals and representatives of voluntary and private organisations. This has implications for social work skills and processes, especially communication.

Point for reflection

For the purposes of these exercises we will concentrate on the situation of Mrs Clark outlined in the chapter and look at this from a variety of perspectives.

- From the perspective of Mrs Clark: think about the situation described in this chapter. Using a systems model, write down or draw a diagram to show potential parts of Mrs Clark's 'system'. Obviously without more detail you will not know precisely who or what is involved, but from your knowledge of similar cases (or from the perspective of older people that you know), think of as many possible parts of the system as possible.

- From the perspective of being a social worker: write down the processes that you would go through if having to deal with the case. When you have done so reflect on which parts of Mrs Clark's system you would be in contact with and in what order.

- From the perspective of a worker with an independent advocacy service for older people: write down the processes that you would go through to fulfil your role as advocate for Mrs Clark. You might want to use some of the website resources to see what they say about advocacy services for older people. When you have done so, reflect on which parts of Mrs Clark's system you would be in contact with.

- Note in what way the different accounts that you have written are similar. In what ways are they different? Do the different roles and tasks involve different parts of Mrs Clark's system?

Putting it into practice

During one day in your practice agency keep a log of your activities. At the end of the day – or another time when you have some space – analyse what you have done.

- How much time did you actually spend face to face with a service user? Would you describe this as working in partnership?
- How much time did you spend acting on behalf of a service user: on the telephone, visiting another agency, looking up information? Would you describe this as advocacy?
- How much time did you spend negotiating with someone: a service user, a manager, a worker from another agency?
- How much time did you spend completing a case record – either manually or on a computer screen – or undertaking some other form of administration?

Look at your results. If you have the opportunity, do this exercise over the period of a week. Consider what it tells you about the way that social work is operating in the agency in which you are undertaking your practice.

Messages from research

The Joseph Rowntree Foundation website http://www.jrf.org.uk/ publications provides a valuable research resource: *Findings from research in social care*. For example, at: http:www.jrf.org.uk/ knowledge/findings/ social care you can find reports such as: *Older People's Perspectives: devising information, advice and advocacy services* by Quinn, A., Snowling, A. and P. Denicolo – a report of research into older people's knowledge and views of advocacy services.

Further resources

Ferguson, I. and Woodward, K. (2009) *Radical Social Work in Practice: Making a difference*. Bristol: Policy Press.
Chapter 6 is an excellent combination of theory, comment and observations from a service user group.

Leadbetter, M. (2002) Chapters on 'Advocacy' and 'Advocacy and empowerment', in R. Adams, Dominelli, L. and Payne, M. (eds) *Social Work: themes, issues and critical debates*. Basingstoke: Palgrave Macmillan.
These are two useful chapters that explore advocacy from the perspective of services users.

McClaughlin, H. (2009) 'What's in a name: "client", "patient", "customer", "consumer", "expert by experience", "service user" – what's next?', *British Journal of Social Work*, 39, pp. 1101–17.
Provides a useful overview and discussion of the implications of the different names used to denote those who are in receipt of social workers' services.

There is a wealth of web pages to be consulted about advocacy services available for user and carer groups: see for example: http://www.ageconcernscotland.org.uk/.

The Scie website on *Adult services: Participation* gives access to information and resources about best practice: http://www.scie.org.uk/adults/participationpub.asp.

Websites such as http://www.partnersinadvocacy.org.uk/ provide information about advocacy services.

CHAPTER 4

Social work processes: communication

Introduction

Communication, especially verbal communication, underpins both the processes of social work discussed so far and the interventions described in the following parts of the text. Social workers might have extensive knowledge and understanding of theories of human behaviour and of a range of possible interventions to help resolve problems, but if they are unable to communicate, to instil confidence, listen and respond appropriately, this knowledge is worthless.

In individual work, most communication takes place in the form of interviews where, either in the office or in the home of the service user, the interchanges are between two people. However, the principles and skills involved in conducting interviews are relevant to family work, groupwork and community work. In all of these situations social workers need to assist people to articulate their needs and to affirm that these needs have been heard, understood and attended to, even if they have not directly been met. This chapter will consider how this can be done in a variety of situations, and when using different social work interventions.

Interviewing

Communication in social work does not happen spontaneously. Interviews are said to be 'conducted' because they are 'conversations with a purpose' (Davies, 1985). Whether the purpose is gathering information for an assessment or encouraging a bereaved person to speak about her/his grief, someone has to help structure the conversation to ensure the purpose is met. Hence the structure of the interview can be as important as the skills used.

In both early referrals and ongoing contact, much depends on the quality of interviewing. Guidance on interviewing is timeless (see texts such as Garrett, 1972; Kadushin, 1972), but obviously interviews have to be relevant to the current context of the service user and changes of emphasis in social work often influence the way interviews are conducted. Therefore, while a social work interview is a conversation with a purpose, it is more than this. An interview is a process in which information about people in their social circumstances, their motivations and their responses in interpersonal relationships can be reflected on, in the light of theory, to help the worker understand the individual in his/her situation, gain relevant information and offer appropriate support.

Only by carefully listening and observing the way that people seek help can there be an effective interpersonal exchange that correctly receives overt and covert messages, decodes them and responds to the various levels of communication. People can say one thing but their behaviour may indicate the opposite. Advanced practitioners, such as those who are expert in family therapy, are able to use the literal message, alongside what is known as the 'metamessage' (that is messages about the message), as part of their interviewing. An illustration of mixed messages is that frequently sent by adolescents to their parents at the crucial stage of leaving home. The bracketed phrase, 'Can I [let you let me] leave?' reveals this. Even if beginners cannot use this level of communication in interviews it is worthwhile at least being able to spot these kinds of underlying motivations.

This is not to say that we should not believe what people say, but recognise that often the messages that are given are complex. One criticism of social workers has been that at times they have used the capacity to interpret messages to disempower those who come to them for assistance. Feminist and radical critiques of social work have parodied such an approach as, 'What you are really saying is ...' suggesting that the worker knows best, will refuse to accept the message that the person is claiming but will impute other meanings. This was a particular source of concern when social work was highly dependent on a psychosocial approach (discussed in the next chapter), and messages were interpreted as having subconscious meanings. Such responses, especially at the beginning of contact, can be off-putting to those who bring problems and issues to the agency. Either they will experience the messages as not being heard, or, if the issue that is being brought is the beginning of a more complex problem, the person might not be ready to share all. Early interpretative approaches may lead to resistance to what might be seen to be an invasion into their privacy. However they can be useful in helping social workers frame their responses, as is discussed later in the chapter.

It is vital that in early interviews the person is helped to say as much as he/she wants to about the situation he/she is bringing to the social worker. Texts about interviewing and research into practice give numerous examples of people making initial contacts with social work agencies, but not being able to share their fears or concerns about the implications of having to make contact. These examples recognise that initial contacts are often made in desperation by service users but are also a screening process for the social work agency. The interactions are therefore crucial: to help the worker establish a beginning relationship with the person seeking help; to inform decisions about whether contact will continue and whether assessment for further services will be undertaken.

Initial interviews

The first meeting between a potential service user and a worker has four major aims:

1. To gather information that will be used jointly in decision making about the nature of the difficulties and how to intervene.
2. To try to secure a 'treatment alliance' whereby the worker conveys a wish to understand the other's thoughts and feelings.
3. To try to include a sense of hopefulness about being able to tackle the circumstances.
4. To demonstrate some of the ways in which the social worker and the service work.

At the beginning of contact, in particular, there is a fine line between inquiry and inquisition; between the need to gain enough information and the need to provide support. Gathering information to help identify whether, and to what extent, help can be offered has to be done without being seen to be inappropriately inquisitive, or not prepared to accept the explanation given. Consider the case of a woman who approaches the social services office for help with day care for her elderly parent. In order to decide whether services can be allocated the worker has to assess both the level of need and the resources that are available. However, in doing this he/she may have to ask about the employment of adults in the family, and caring and other responsibilities of all concerned. Ultimately, there will also be questions about financial circumstances. Such information gathering has to be conducted in ways which do not invoke feelings of guilt, or make the woman feel that she is becoming a 'client' of the agency, in the worst sense of the word.

Situations that involve those who are reluctant participants, that is, offenders, or parents who may be suspected of abusing their children, bring other dilemmas. In the former, information has to be gathered for the purpose of assessment about the level of motivation for compliance with supervision or a community sentence, while it is recognised that a driving factor may be the desire to avoid a custodial sentence. When accusations and allegations of abuse have to be investigated, or suspicions followed up, very sensitive information has to be acquired. But it must be remembered that the person being investigated may be innocent, and even if he or she is not, he/she will need a continuing relationship with a social work agency in order to ensure the appropriate outcome for all involved.

When individuals have come of their own accord to the agency, they are motivated by all sorts of factors which can lead to a range of responses. For example, many people are quite satisfied with the first session and decide that they do not require further assistance or they are so overwhelmed by the intensity or chronic nature of their problems that they cannot use the help that is offered. Others are not ready to commit themselves to ongoing intervention, while a high proportion of people prefer to ask for help on an as-needed basis rather than have a regular series of meetings. This might be because they do not want to be seen as a 'client' or 'service user', which carries stigma. Such responses are to do with society's negative perceptions of social work, which also leads to assumptions that only limited help can be offered or that social workers are merely gatekeepers of resources.

In initial interviews for community care services the worker might well have to operate eligibility criteria either for services or, as in the case of those who might qualify for personalised budgets, resources to purchase services. In these circumstances it is possible that at the end of the interview the worker has to inform the person seeking help or support that services are not available. This may be because he or she has come to the wrong agency, and needs to be referred to a benefits agency or to a health service. Alternatively it may be because he/she does not fit the eligibility criteria, or it is thought that the problem is not acute or sufficiently chronic to warrant further assessment at this stage. In these circumstances the person has to be given clear and full information about why the decision is made. This has to be done in such a way that people feel validated and not rejected. In circumstances where people are involved in caring, it is likely that the situation will deteriorate and at some point in the future another referral will be made. It is therefore necessary to ensure that the person will feel able to come back to the agency.

There are ways of conducting an initial interview that are more likely to establish a favourable climate for a purposeful alliance. These involve ensuring that there is congruence, that is, agreement between worker and service user about expectations of what can be done, and being open and honest about what cannot be done. From the outset all parties should be aware of why they are meeting (or talking). Successful interviews do not merely depend on content (what was said) or whether the service user got what was asked for. A significant outcome for the first interview is for the worker to be perceived as someone who is able to understand the concerns, how the person feels about his/her difficulties and is open about both the agency and the worker's own role within it. Additionally the worker will have demonstrated some of the basic values of social work, including acceptance and a non-judgemental attitude.

Skills in interviewing

Early accounts of social work identified basic skills in interviewing that involve ten principles:

1. Letting the interviewee know how much time there is.
2. Starting where the client is in his/her understanding of the situation.
3. Trying to be sympathetic so as to help make the atmosphere a relaxed one.
4. Trying to see things through the other person's eyes.
5. Knowing the danger of passing judgement rather than acceptance.
6. Developing social skills such as smiling to help open up communication at the outset.
7. Avoiding questions that can be answered 'yes' or 'no'.
8. Not putting answers in the client's mouth.
9. Not probing too deeply too quickly.
10. Learning to cope with silences (which are usually the interviewee's best thinking times). (Davies, 1985)

These 'principles' are based on core social work values such as respect for persons (Biestek, 1957; Banks, 2006) and 'starting where the client is'. The skill required in an interview is in how that respect is communicated, irrespective of the circumstances or content of the interview. However, this does not mean that the interview has to be aimless: respect also requires that the person is important enough for the worker to have prepared for the interview. Preparation involves understanding what happens in interviews.

Structure

Each interview has a focus, such as an exploration of someone's financial needs, illnesses, offences, relationships. Every interview also ought to have a structure: a beginning, middle and end. However, there is circularity in the interviewing process if it is to make sense to the person being interviewed and provide the necessary information. The person bringing the problem or issue will set the initial agenda, but the interviewer asking more questions helps to develop themes. Appropriate questions might lead to further information and other avenues to be explored. At the close of the interview, the interviewer should ensure that the original topic is returned to, and reviewed in the light of the information that has emerged during the interview. These stages are discussed in the next chapter in relation to Egan's work on counselling, but are relevant to some degree in all interviews.

The first words at the beginning of any encounter are often quite significant, for example, 'My doctor thought that you could help me' suggests reluctance on the part of the person coming to the agency. Equally the last things said could reveal what attitude the person leaves with, for instance, 'I think I can cope now I've got the information' recognises that the person leaves with reassurance as well as information.

The language that is used often reveals emotions as, of course, do the bodily positions and non-verbal gestures displayed during the interviews. In both single interviews and in a series of interviews, references to difficulties may be returned to. Repetition or even denial that something is worrying may give clues to helping. Other indicators are inconsistencies and gaps, for instance mentioning one parent but never the other one, or concealed meanings such as the sexually abused client who fears interference (being interfered with?). Sudden changes in conversation topics may indicate material that is too painful, or that the person may have made associations between ideas which are not obvious to the worker. All of these are important.

Questioning

As has been said, as interviews proceed they have to achieve a fine balance in order to gather necessary information. This is especially so at the beginning of any contact and in the processes of assessment, review and quality assurance. Information can be gathered by observation and listening, but the most common way is to ask questions which get at both facts and feelings. As Chapter 2 discussed, the use of schedules and pro forma to log information increases workers need to be skilled in asking questions appropriately in order to get this information sensitively. For example, an interviewer who poses questions accusingly or in a suspicious tone rather than in an interested and friendly way will arouse fear and antagonism. The wording of a question in this respect is less important than the manner and tone in which it is put. Try asking the question 'Are you looking for work?' a number of times putting emphasis on a different word each time you say it.

Open questions

Obviously questions have to be asked to get some information, especially when it has not been forthcoming in the interview. A general rule for social work is that more information is gleaned and more is learned about people's reactions by asking open questions. These are questions that require more than the answer 'yes' or 'no'. The question, 'Do you have any children?' will elicit the answer 'yes' or 'no'; the question, 'How many children do you have?' will get information about the number of children, and might also encourage the person to give details about them, thus avoiding the need for further questions about the sex and age of the children. It is often recommended that the 5WH (Why, What, Who, Where, When and How) are useful to help us think about open questions. A blend of enquiries that address these areas will reveal a lot of fundamental information: 'Why is this a problem?' 'When did it start?' 'Who could help?' 'What needs to happen?' 'How do you think we can help?' Obviously these would not be asked all at once, or in quick succession!

Careful thought needs to be given even in the use of open questions. The overuse of the question 'Why?' might seem to imply that someone should explain their behaviour, and cause defences to go up. In any event, people often do not know 'Why?' and may be seeking help to understand themselves and their situation more clearly. A 'What?' alternative is preferable and may reveal information useful to all involved in the interchange, as happened when a worker, instead of asking an elderly person why she was afraid to go out, asked what she thought might happen if she did. This reframing of questions has become particularly significant in solution-focused approaches discussed in Chapter 8.

Probing questions

Skilful use of questions is sometimes overlooked in social work, as if it is something anyone can do. As an alternative to questions to collect information that appears to have value only to the organisation (which increases resistance, for example in involuntary clients in probation), probing questions are a way of actually starting off processes of change. It is worth studying the range of good questioning techniques that can help others identify their experience, raise consciousness, solve problems and so on (see Lefevre 2010 for a discussion). What are called 'naïve' questions can be used to understand how people who are overwhelmed by their situation perceive it and to encourage a change in that perception. Reporter-type questions can sometimes achieve the same goal, as can the devil's advocate approach. Here the respondent is intentionally confronted with the arguments of opponents in order to trigger a change. Other ways of employing questions that hold the germs of possible change involve taking a one-down stance by saying, 'I could be wrong but ...'; 'I wonder ...' or, 'I don't quite understand ...', all of which stimulate people to step outside of their usual frame of reference to consider new possibilities, without the worker dragging out information.

Asking too many questions can be like an interrogation: asking too few questions may leave relevant features hidden. The pace at which questions are put needs to be the service user's, otherwise more might be revealed than the person intended, resulting in annoyance or reluctance to return to the agency. However, it is sometimes possible to assist people to say what they want to, or give you the information you need to be able to help them by a process of *funnelling*. This encourages people to speak quite generally about a subject, encouraged by the prompt to 'Tell me about ...' You can then ask them to give a specific example of what they are talking about, and then focus on that example, but also check out how frequently such events or experiences occur.

Another general guideline is to log awkward moments and return to them later when the service user can cope with a specific question, perhaps acknowledging the awkwardness and underlining an earlier question by asking it again. All of these ways of helping people both describe their situation and to think about changing it reminds us that questioning techniques and other aspects of communication underpin all interventions, not just assessment.

Circular questioning

Another style of asking good questions is that known as 'circular questioning'. Developed within family therapy it assesses family functioning and interaction by asking one member of the family to comment on the relationship or behaviour of two other members. Thus, 'When your mother tries to get Andrew to go to school, what does your grandmother do?' and, 'Who do you think is closer to your father, your sister or your brother?' and so on. Circular questioning highlights different viewpoints, giving feedback to everyone present while introducing new information about how each third party views relations between the others (Lask, 2010).

Hypothetical questions, starting with 'What if?', are additionally revealing for all, as are those that ask people to describe their ideal solution. This can give clues to people's goals and the way in which work might move forward. It is now associated with the 'magic bullet' of solution-focused work discussed in Chapter 8. Such questions also provide a challenge to people's assumptions. An adolescent boy who is being fostered, but is in conflict with his family and threatening to leave home, could be encouraged to explore: 'What if you left home, what do you think would happen?' This might enable him to explain his worries or fears – perhaps that his foster parents did not (and would not) care about what happened to him.

Problem-posing questions are preferable to responding with ready answers that undermine the competence of those that are in the situation. People often have their own ideas that can be 'unlocked'. For example, a despairing group of homeless people at a drop-in centre who said 'We can't change their policies' were induced to rethink their powerlessness by a worker who asked, 'Who are they, and what do we know of their policies?' In sum, asking good questions saves time, helps to engage rather than alienate service users, and can be a tool for beginning to change a situation.

Avoidance

It is very common amongst inexperienced workers to avoid asking questions for a variety of reasons: avoidance of probing questions can occur when there are hints at more complicated issues. Failing to pursue some areas in an interview might be related to needing to protect ourselves from pain or fear of unearthing material that is threatening or distressing; over-cautiousness or reticence can be a hindrance. For example, if someone hints that he or she is so depressed that he/she wonders if life is worth living and then quickly moves on to another subject, it might be worthwhile coming back to that idea again later. This can be done by saying something like, 'Can you tell me more about that?' or 'I'm not sure I understood earlier when you said ...' This allows for elaboration if the person wants this; it also lets the worker check out perceptions, and it conveys to the service user that the worker can cope with the 'unacceptable' thoughts and feelings.

Avoidance can also occur when suspicions are raised about behaviour and attitudes that are unacceptable, inappropriate or even illegal. This is particularly sensitive in relationships where the worker has a responsibility for monitoring behaviour. For example, the requirements in criminal justice work to confront offending behaviour, or for childcare workers to ensure the protection of

children, can precipitate dilemmas for workers if they receive information in interviews that clearly indicates inappropriate or unacceptable behaviour. In these circumstances, there is sometimes an
appeal to confidentiality, an expectation that the worker will not
act on the information. It is therefore important to be clear about
the parameters; if the person then chooses to reveal information
he/she does so knowing that the worker will have to act upon it.

Early responses to dealing with issues of race were for workers
to avoid challenging black and ethnic minority people in the same
way as white people might be challenged. It is appropriate to challenge behaviour that is deemed to be unacceptable, as long as
workers check out that their judgement is not framed by unfair
stereotypes or the application of cultural norms, which may lead
them to misinterpret certain behaviour and/or attitudes (Bhatti-
Sinclair, 2011). Equally, working with assumptions that all service
users are in heterosexual relationships might avoid issues of sexual
orientation that might be important for individuals.

Responding

Interviewing is not just a one-way process; it is not just about
asking questions and listening to the answers. Asking questions can
be a way of responding – but there other ways of communicating
appropriate responses. Most people, when they listen, give some
indication of the fact that they have heard; saying nothing can
appear uninterested or even hostile. There are ways to demonstrate
that you are listening: sitting attentively or nodding at appropriate
points are two ways, but much more significant are the responses
that are made. Five types of responses have been identified, not all
of which are good practice.

1. *Evaluative* responses are those that say how you judge the
   person, or what is being told to you. Many remarks in
   ordinary conversation carry evaluative overtones. These are
   to be avoided. Good listeners will learn to accept people, and
   hear information without passing judgement about what
   they hear.
2. *Interpretative* responses analyse what the person has said, and
   give it new meaning. This is often an intellectual response, and
   can be attractive to students who are encouraged to link their
   practice to theory. Almost always, interpretative responses

lead away from what the person is saying, but represent what is going on in the listener's mind. Interpretations should be used sparingly – even when we are asked directly what we think.

3. *Sympathetic* responses might seem appropriate if people are sad or upset, or what they are talking about seems painful. However, there is a danger that in expressing sympathy you are reacting to how you think you might be feeling in the circumstances. In social work accurate empathy not sympathy is necessary. This involves listening to, and accepting, the emotions that people are expressing, however unexpected they might seem in the circumstances. If you name an emotion for someone, you might stop that person being able to express what he or she really feels, because he/she thinks their emotion is 'inappropriate'.

4. *Probing* responses are those that seek more detail about what is said, but often they are based on the listener's interpretation of the situation and seeking confirmation of this. As has been said, a good use of probing is when people are encouraged to explore their own feelings about what they are saying. This helps us to understand what they are experiencing.

5. *Understanding* responses are those needed to be a good listener. There are three kinds of understanding responses:

   • *Reflecting:* this is usually demonstrated by repeating what someone has said – reflecting it back to them. This is not done merely in parrot fashion, but more as an echo of his/her thoughts. It acts as a prompt enabling that person to change or clarify the words that he/she has used and encouraging him/her to say more without directing or probing. It is also a clear indicator that you are actively hearing what the person says.

   • *Paraphrase:* if you repeat back what someone has said, perhaps using different words, or joining together two or three things that he/she has said without changing the meaning, this is paraphrasing. It is important if summarising a complicated set of events or feelings that you do not interpret or evaluate them. It is also necessary to check out with the person that what you have paraphrased is accurate.

   • *Feedback:* this is given when you want to indicate that you have heard accurately what has been said, and that you accept the person, whatever the emotions expressed or information given. So, for example, it is possible to tell a bereaved person that it is alright to feel angry with the person who has died, if that is the emotion that has been expressed. But it is always important to check out with the person that you have fed back accurately.

The 'techniques' described above are those that can be used in most situations that social workers deal with. However, in different parts of this book, methods of intervention are described that require specific approaches. For example, solution-focused therapy (Chapter 8) requires the worker to identify the 'miracle' question while motivational interviewing in cognitive behavioural work (Chapter 9) depends on an established series of questions. What is interesting is that the early writings about what was then called casework took from counselling an overview of the kinds of communication in social work. They identified two main procedures that can inform responses in social work: sustaining and modifying (Hollis, 1964).

Sustaining procedures: are those techniques familiar to practitioners who talk about 'offering support' or 'building a relationship'. They include:

- *Ventilation* – involves facilitating people to unburden feelings and thoughts which allows them to concentrate on problem solving.
- *Realistic reassurance* – by keeping the person in touch with actuality, not promising what cannot be done, keeping an appraisal of external facts to the forefront.
- *Acceptance* – is a basic social work value (Banks, 2006). Demonstrating it by different ways of communicating allows the person to acknowledge 'bad' feelings and lessens self-criticism, overwork, rigidity, shame at having a problem, and so on.
- *Logical discussion* – gives the worker scope to assess someone's ability to reason and confront reality without needing to retreat into fantasy, symptoms of physical illness, pessimism and so on.
- *Demonstrating behaviour* – whereby the worker models coping. This has been developed further in processes of pro-social modelling (see Chapter 9). However in all communication the worker needs to demonstrate he/she can be trusted and depended upon to be able to tolerate frustration,

set limits, keep perspective – and this helps the service user to observe and perhaps internalise these – and try them out in the interview.

- *Giving information* – increases motivation and problem solving because it helps to separate the facts of what is 'inside' the person, their fears and misperceptions, and 'outside' in relation to facts and resources.

- *Offering advice and guidance* – usually it is not good practice to rush to offer advice and guidance but, in psychosocial terms, it can enlarge understanding. It is sustaining because it gives the service user support and enables them to keep control: reducing doubt and fear of the unknown introduces hope and assists capacity for reflection, adaptation and readiness to cope.

- *Environmental manipulation* – this is a 'technical' term from Hollis (1964) which is now referred to as 'working with the environment' or the 'social'. It includes actually doing things on behalf of, or with, service users: helping with rehousing, money and/or advocacy. By helping or trying to obtain needed resources the worker shares the burden of handling practical problems. Reducing anxiety increases self-confidence and helps reduce feelings of shame and guilt; or anger.

Modifying procedures: these also aim to reduce outer pressures but at the same time try to increase awareness of how an individual's personality, reactions and behaviour can influence situations. In social work terms this involves the person gaining insight and includes:

- *Reflective communications* – in any social work intervention reflection aids self-understanding by helping individuals consider in a new light their opinions, attitudes, behaviour, present feelings, past traumas, early life experiences. In counselling the person goes on to use the relationship with the worker as a way of changing their perceptions and/or behaviour.

- *Confrontation techniques* – include pointing out patterns of thinking, feeling and doing that are perhaps not helpful. Confrontation may show how the service user responds in particular ways in their relationships, using an example of the client–worker relationship itself. For example, a person who has had bad experience of dependency could have difficulty accepting anything that the worker says.

- *Clarification techniques* – involve the use of interpretations to point out, for example, when a person's use of defence mechanisms is getting in the way of change, making him/her resistant. For example 'Whenever we get around to talking about your father you change the topic, I wonder why that is?'
- *Interpretation* – can be a major procedure and might be necessary when symptoms are used as a diversion away from painful conflicts in life and in an individual's inner world. Usually it requires an observation that helps to link present circumstances in someone's life 'out there' to the feelings that they have 'in here' (that is, the relationship with the helper) and to what went on 'back there' (the past). An example is a person who is unable to stay in any job without becoming resentful and challenging towards female managers. The worker might interpret it: 'You say you get anxious with women in authority. I remember you saying your mother was the boss at home. I wonder if you feel worried now because I am a woman who seems to be telling you what to do?'

  This kind of interpretation can be questioned because (a) insight does not necessarily lead to change; and (b) it gives the worker a great deal of power. However these methods are often no more than a reflective discussion of making sense with and for the individual and they can help answer questions such as 'Why am I like this?' The aim is that the person might see things a little differently and feel that he/she has more control over his/her problems in the present.

This detailed discussion of the structure, process and content of interviews indicates that each interview needs to be both prepared for and reflected upon. In training this can involve reviewing aspects of the content of each encounter, if possible via a detailed record or (as in certain agencies such as those using family therapies) by means of a video recording. While difficult to follow in day-to-day practice, it is important to build in some reflective mechanisms (see Chapter 5). Such reflections should include an awareness of the powerful role that the interviewer plays both in helping the person explore the issues fully in a way that he/she wants to and in the potential to block communication. They can help identify both progress that has been made and barriers to communication.

Barriers to communication

Barriers to communication can come from a number of sources. There are circumstances where verbal communication is not appropriate or the most helpful means of intervening. There may be reasons why individual service users have difficulty communicating, for example, some people with learning difficulties (Cambridge and Forrester-Jones, 2003) or those with hearing impairment (Young *et al.*, 2000). However, there are also some overarching difficulties in communication not related to the specific needs of certain service users.

Sometimes students are daunted by the things they have to think about when undertaking interviews. They become even more anxious when they encounter people who are uncooperative and who, despite saying that they want help, seem to do all that they can to block it. Often the reason for this is about the balances within the interviewing situation. Approaching a stranger for help could be an occasion for shame, high expectations, sense of failure and an admission of dependency – all of which can cause resentment. The worker does not have to reveal intimate, embarrassing or frightening facts about her or himself and so there is understandable reluctance and anger on the part of the interviewee, which may, indeed, remind him/her of times past when similar interpersonal contacts proved unhelpful. It might also be a reminder of the power balances within the situation. It is vital that the worker remains sensitive to these power balances throughout any interview. This is not to say that interviewers should never exercise power – but that they need to know when they are doing it, why they are doing it and why it is justified.

One way of addressing power imbalances is to eliminate some of the barriers to communication that can contribute to misinterpretations and misunderstandings. Attention must be paid to issues of diversity when undertaking interviews. Stereotyping can lead to inaccurate assumptions that block the individual and this can create defences. Assuming that because someone is black, or middle class, or an asylum seeker he or she will have certain characteristics encourages premature judgements and hasty conclusions. Also, there should be no automatic assumption about a person's sexual orientation. People are too complex, subtle and dynamic to sum up rapidly, and rapid judgements can create difficult dynamics. On the one hand, being antagonistic because someone is aggressive can exacerbate situations in ways that are not helpful for the user and could ultimately lead to risks for the worker. On the other hand, warming to someone because of their charm, ability to verbalise and their seeming cooperation can lead to a false sense of positiveness, to collusion and denial of significant factors (for example child abuse or domestic violence).

Using jargon or technical terms is another obvious obstacle to good interviewing; it distances worker and client. Using the service user's own words and phrases is often useful. As has been said already, it demonstrates that you are listening attentively, clarifies understanding and at the same time conveys acceptance and respect for his/her way of putting things. However, it is also important not to be seen to be condescending.

When working with black and ethnic minority service users, it is important that workers acknowledge there might be the need for special attention to other issues of diversity. An awareness that religion and culture can create different expectations is important in communication and should make workers alert to questions such as: who conducts the interview (issues of gender can be crucial), who attends the interview (if a Muslim woman has to be accompanied, what is the relationship to the person who is present), where and when the interview is held (recognising the significance of different times of the day, days of the week and months in the year). Where there are language differences, then it is vital that appropriate attention is paid to working with interpreters.

Using interpreters

Changing policies towards refugees and asylum seekers (Newbigging et al., 2010) and greater mobility within the European workforce mean social workers are increasingly required to work with people for whom either English is not their first language, or they do not speak it at all and therefore an interpreter is required. In using interpreters, it is important to demonstrate respect by understanding attitudes to asking for help and about social work in the person's culture or country of origin. It might seem obvious that identifying correctly which language a person speaks is fundamental, but it is not always easy when there are different versions and dialects.

There are other barriers in the case of asylum seekers where the fact that a social worker is an 'agent of the state' might have particular connotations. This has implications for who is asked to provide the interpretation. Working through children or relatives is not acceptable, as this denies the person confidentiality and constrains the information that can be given.

The interpreter is a conduit linking interviewer and interviewee, and thus careful preparation of the interpreter for this role is necessary, emphasising confidentiality, neutrality, conveying the emotional tone of the interview and transmitting accurately what is being communicated. It is crucial that interpreters are trained and qualified and fluent in the relevant language and vocabulary to be able to explain procedures and rights and to discuss interpersonal issues that might be highly sensitive. The use of interpreters means that the person giving personal information has to give it to more than one person. The trained interpreter offers objectivity in a way that using a family member or friends does not. However the interpreter may still be experienced by the person needing help as in some way judging him or her. This might be particularly so where the crisis or problem has been precipitated by cultural dilemmas. For example, Muslim women may feel reluctant to speak about domestic violence to an interpreter, because of cultural expectations of the role of women within marriage. It is therefore vital that the interpreter's presence is accepted and there is a commitment to confidentiality from everyone (see Robinson, 1998; Alexander *et al.*, 2004).

Agencies should fulfil their obligations to offer services to non-English-speaking clients by recruiting and training interpreters to function within that role, but this is not unproblematic (Newbigging *et al.*, 2010). However many health and social care organisations have developed specific policies and guidance on using interpreters and it is vital that all workers are familiar with these – and raise questions if they do not exist.

Interviewing children

Interviewing children and adolescents requires particular skills. Specialist literature for teaching and learning communication skills (Lefevre, 2010) is available and should be consulted, and practice gained through experience, courses and maybe micro-skills teaching via video and live supervision. Interviewers who are skilled in adult work can find it hard to communicate with children because of a tendency to concentrate too much on the formal elements of the interviewing task. For instance, using questions is different with children with whom, in fact-finding, one may need to be quite specific and direct. Letting the child talk freely while gaining facts takes expertise. Gaining cooperation, timing, overcoming confusion, managing hostility, being spontaneous, getting the right surroundings, communicating through what Lefevre calls the 'hundred languages of childhood' (2010, p. 169) is vital. As she points out children are not always able to name their emotions and helping them do this by using 'third things' (toys and analogies), encouraging expression through art work, stories, music and role play can be creative. Using touch is also a possibility but has to be used with caution (Lynch and Garrett, 2010). Workers need to ensure that the methods used are appropriate for the particular child – ensuring, among other things, age and cultural appropriateness.

At the outset of becoming a social worker it is difficult because many of these 'techniques' might be being used at the same time – and it is hard to remember everything. Often it feels as if concentrating on what you think you must and must not do gets in the way of what is important – letting people feel that they are valued and that you are concerned about them. In the short term, you are unlikely to cause too much harm as long as you concentrate on listening and do not make precipitous interventions, give false reassurance or make unrealistic promises. In many cases there will be the opportunity to reflect on what you have heard, and what you have said, and to think about how future interviews can build on this. With this careful reflection and the opportunity to think about what worked in terms of what you did and said, there is the potential to become skilled. However no matter how many years' experience you have and how skilled you feel, it is always necessary to build in time to consider the content and process of interviews. This will not only help to synthesise information that might be used in assessment but will also help inform decisions about what method of intervention is most appropriate for the situation.

Conclusion

This chapter has focused on some of the basic skills required to facilitate communication in social work. It has underlined that effective communication is vital for good social work practice, and that it operates at all parts of the social work process. Importantly, effective communication has to be consistent with the value base of social work, that is, it has to reflect respect for persons and be non-oppressive and non-discriminatory. As will be seen in the next section, specific types of intervention based on different theoretical approaches to social problems all draw on these basic skills of communication, but develop them in different ways – depending on the function and purpose of the particular intervention.

Point for reflection

This chapter is very much an introduction to communication, focusing on interviews. Now that you have read the chapter it would be useful to reflect on it using the following:

• Write down your three main concerns about undertaking interviews, based on what you have read and your practice experience if you have any.
• Write down the three main 'lessons' you have learnt from reading it.

Is there any mismatch? Does the chapter address your concerns or are you still looking for guidance and reassurance? It would not be unusual if you are – in fact it indicates that you want to do your best in communication.

Hopefully the exercise below and the resources identified (especially the SCIE resources) will help. However the best way to build up skills is to practice, and to reflect on your experiences.

Putting it into practice

Practising communication skills is difficult on one's own, and it is better to do this in group settings. Also, the use of video and other feedback mechanisms is helpful, as long as the feedback is given in a helpful and constructive manner – we are all nervous when we are observed, and it is very easy to point out where things could be done better.

However there are some exercises that can be done without the aid of technology:

1 Listen to conversations. If interviews are conversations with a purpose, it is revealing to listen to how unpurposeful seemingly aimless conversations can be. Without being too nosey or obtrusive listen in to snatches of conversation (between two people – not the one-sided ones on mobile phones!) There might also be something to learn from watching reality TV! Note the way that people do/do not listen to each other, how the conversation moves in unexpected directions and to what extent an individual does/does not dominate the conversation.

2 Now focus on yourself. Start listening to your own everyday conversations. This is not to suggest that you should be using social work skills in all your conversations. However it is useful to listen to oneself in different circumstances and with different people, and again to observe whether you get to say what you want in conversations, whether you really listen to friends, colleagues and acquaintances. Are there some people with whom you have conversations where you feel more involved/engaged? If so, ask yourself 'Why'?

3 Use the media. Listen to different interviewing techniques on the radio and the television. Note those techniques that you feel are effective, and write down what it is about the technique that is effective. Be clear about what 'effectiveness' is. Note what aspects of these interviews you find unacceptable. Why? Are there any aspects of particular interviewer's technique that you might adopt? If so what, and why?

Messages from research

Cambridge, P. and Forrester-Jones, R. (2003) 'Using individualised communication for interviewing people with intellectual disability: a case study of user-centred research', *Journal of Intellectual & Developmental Disability* (1), pp. 5–23. Although not directly about social work practice this article discusses communication methods used to enable people with intellectual disability to participate in outcome and quality of life research.

Further resources

Lefevre, M. (2010) *Communicating with Children and Young People Making a Difference*. Bristol: Policy Press.
This is an excellent text that gives background theory on communication and specific attention to communicating with children and young people.

Lishman, J. (1995) *Communication in Social Work*. Basingstoke: BASW/Macmillan.
A comprehensive text that is an important resource for social work students and practitioners, and discusses written and verbal communication in specific social work processes.

Robinson, L. (1998) *Race: communication and the caring professions.*
Buckingham: Open University Press.
An important text in that it focuses solely on the way health and
social care professions communicate with black and ethnic minority
service users and carers.

The Social Care Institute for Excellence (Scie) website has a wealth of
resources including audio, video and interactive technology to do
with good communication skills and how to use these:
http://www.scie.org.uk/publications/elearning/cs/index.asp.

CHAPTER 5

Social work processes: reflection and review

CHAPTER OVERVIEW
- Reflective practice
- Review stages in social work
- Endings

In the previous chapters mention has been made of both reflection and review. This final chapter in the section on processes explores these in more detail. Both should underpin all social work practice. The difference between them is to do with both timing and the processes involved. At an organisational level, review provides an overview of social work intervention: it can be a one-off event or it can occur periodically. At the level of individual work, it occurs at identified stages within a period of intervention. Reflection is a process which is ongoing throughout all social work intervention and beyond.

Reflective practice

Reflective practice has been discussed in the context of assessment but it is also core to all social work interventions. Trevithick describes interventions in social work as purposeful actions under-taken by professionals in a given situation based on knowledge and understanding acquired and skills learned and values adopted: 'interventions are knowledge, skills, understanding and values in action' (2005a, p. 66). In order to achieve such synthesis, workers need to engage in reflective practice.

A number of different terms, including reflexive; reflective prac-tice and critical reflection, are used in the literature (Fook and Gardner, 2007) but in social work all relate to the process of what we will call reflective practice. The process first became popular in social work through the work of Schon (1987), who explored how to educate and enable practitioners to use both their knowledge and experience to inform their work and develop expertise.

Terminology can be problematic, but it is also crucial. For example *reflexive* can imply something that is spontaneous and automatic – knee jerk. In Chapter 1 we considered that social work is sometimes accused of being just 'common sense', which can involve knee-jerk reactions. Therefore it is important to demonstrate that social work is more reflective, drawing on theory and research. *Reflective* can indicate contemplative and meditative approaches – musing. However in discussions about the development of social work as a profession that have argued for social workers to have better qualifications and more theoretical knowledge, it has been suggested that people in crises or with multiple problems cannot wait for social workers to muse on all the possible alternatives for action. But, if reflection is built into all practice, it does not have to slow the process of helping. Having said that, uncritical interventions, those that are not thought through, might be unhelpful and sometimes harmful as many child abuse tragedies illustrate.

Research into professional practice (Benner, 1984; Fook *et al.*, 2000; DoH, 2008a) has shown that expertise in social work is achieved when practitioners can react spontaneously while drawing on their accumulated knowledge and experience. This could be seen as reflexivity based on reflection or as Schon (1987) puts it, reflection in action.

However the interpretation of reflexivity as 'turning back on itself' has led to suggestions that reflexivity requires practitioners to look inwards and outwards. This is necessary when looking at our own reactions to the situations with which we deal, but also how we make sense of them using theory. Taylor and White (2000) argue that practitioners must engage actively with what they read, subject it to scrutiny and recognise how it suggests different understandings of a situation. This can be seen in the reflective exercises that occur at the end of the chapters in this book. Taylor and White (2000) use the verb 'practising' (reflexivity), as opposed to the noun (reflexive) 'practice'. Reflexivity they argue has to be 'done', it does not simply exist.

For Trevithick (2005a), reflective practice involves both critical thinking and practice wisdom. In some ways practice wisdom is the 'common sense' of social work practice. It is the wisdom derived from experience and personal knowledge about what works in a particular situation. However, critical thinking requires the practitioner to have an open mind when first encountering situations and to 'check out' whether the common sense or knee-jerk reaction is the right one. For example frequently in reviews of child abuse cases social workers have reported that the child 'seemed' happy and there was no need to investigate further. The knee-jerk reaction is not to upset child and parent by being more inquisitive or inspectorial. However the bruises hidden by chocolate, the appalling living conditions go undetected and have, on occasions, led to tragic deaths of children.

The 'avoidance' that might be perceived as influencing a worker's reluctance to investigate such situations too closely is an important focus for reflection for Fook (2002). She argues that critical reflection involves the identification of deep-seated assumptions and therefore must incorporate an understanding of personal experiences within social, cultural and structural contexts. Ultimately through critical reflection especially about the social world and the individual person's connection with it, the individual and the worker have a better sense of how that world is constructed. This insight should enable the person to become more empowered and able to act within and upon her or his social world (Fook and Askeland, 2007). Critical reflection can be instrumental in helping practitioners understand what informs their knee-jerk reactions, and therefore raising their awareness of how they might react in certain situations. It can also help service users to understand their own responses to their situation.

Practitioners are encouraged to reflect on their experience using critical incident analysis in a workshop setting to help develop professional growth and social change (Fook and Askeland, 2007; Fook and Gardner, 2007). This growth is necessary because of practitioners' involvement in their work: 'we are experiencing the situation we seek to understand and we are part of the intervention we are involved in providing' (Trevithick, 2005a, p. 252).

This involvement of the practitioner suggests a level of subjectivity that has been seen to be at odds with developing requirements for evidence- or research-based practice. However, the argument that the use of 'evidence' gives an unbiased, objective basis for social work has been questioned (Healy, 2005; Orme and Shemmings, 2010). Healy (2005) suggests evidence-based practice and reflective practice have been unhelpfully polarised in social work. The former is associated with the need for empirical evidence while the latter argues for recognition of practitioners' lived experience. She recognises the danger that relying on, or prioritising, experiential knowledge might mean that practitioners fail to fully utilise formal theories. This could mean that at worst they rely on knee-jerk reactions while at best they end up 'reinventing the wheel rather than building and developing existing theories' (Healy, 2005, p. 101). The potential of critical reflection is not that it overthrows or throws out all other understandings of theory, but that it challenges assumptions that only certain theories are valid. It does not mean that only one form of knowledge, that is, either theoretical or practitioner and service user knowledge, is valid; it accepts that all have a contribution to make to understanding situations, and therefore constructing theory about them. This synthesis, of different knowledge, called 'reflexive practice' by Taylor and White (2000), involves the iteration of empirical knowledge with experiential knowledge; that is, they both inform each other and each is developed and improved by the knowledge gained from the other. Such an approach is now so accepted in social work that it provides the rationale for some textbooks (see Cree and Myers, 2008) and is addressed in specific training programmes (Fook and Gardner, 2007).

While critical reflection is required throughout social work interventions to ensure best practice, it should also be undertaken in conjunction with more formal approaches to understanding and explaining the situations in which social workers are intervening. This is the process of review.

Review

Review is the infrastructure for social work and occurs at a variety of levels. Perhaps the most formal and most high-profile reviews are those that are instigated at the request of governments, usually after some tragedy or perceived mismanagement. Sometimes referred to as 'enquiries' these reviews aim to investigate the practice of individuals and organisations and identify where improvements can be made. As such, these are sometimes experienced negatively by practitioners. Other more positive (in terms of how they present social work) examples of such meta-reviews include the 21st Century Review of Social Work in Scotland (Scottish Executive, 2006a) and the Munro Review of Child Protection in England (Department for Education, 2011). Although both arose out of challenges to the profession of social work, they sought to find ways of positively examining the role and task of social work and to create the conditions that enable professionals to make the best judgements.

The second level of review is that which involves organisational review. Healy (2005) points out that social work is a negotiated activity between institutional context, formal purpose, professional base and frameworks for practice. Because of the contentious nature of social work's place in society, this negotiated activity is subject to review. Policy initiatives such as *Best Value* and legislation such as the *Care Standards Act* (2000) require a form of review which can be experienced by practitioners as part of the blame culture (Bell, 2005) and have been referred to as 'evaluation with a big E' (Shaw and Shaw, 1997).

Such reviews, sometimes called overviews, are ultimately the responsibility of the organisation: 'Social services departments have lead responsibility for ensuring these reviews take place within the prescribed time scales' (DoH, 2000c, p. 65). However the performance of the organisation depends on every staff member following best practice, which includes ensuring that procedures are followed at all levels.

Linked to such quality assurance reviews is a third level of review and involves activities which are part of a general set of national frameworks developed to set national standards and identify key interventions for the relevant services (Bell, 2005; Hafford-Letchfield, 2007). Examples of such reviews are those that have been established by policies such as the *Framework of Assessment for Children in Need and their Families* (DoH, 2000c) and the *Care Programme Approach* (CPA) for people in the mental health system. Both involve critical and timely judgement about what is happening in a situation.

The framework for the assessment of children in need and their families (see Chapter 2) was developed to provide 'a systematic way of analysing, understanding and recording what is happening to children and young people within their families and the wider context of the community in which they live' (DoH 2000c, p. viii). One aim of the assessment framework is to identify early indicators of risk but also to identify different types and levels of need and ensure appropriate and timely responses. Central to the process are the principles of safeguarding those within the systems. Therefore it is not appropriate for work to continue without identified points at which it can be appraised or reviewed.

Another example of how such processes can be systematised is the introduction of Independent Reviewing Officers (IROs) through the Review of Children's Cases (Amendment) (England) Regulations 2004. This recognises that children, whose interests had been protected during care proceedings, needed independent safeguarding from the occasional acute failings of the care system as identified in some enquiries. It has the effect of returning responsibility for monitoring of children's wellbeing in the care system to the social work profession with the aim of avoiding the chronic failings of what has been termed 'drift'.

Such systems also recognise that the best interests of the child have to be recognised by focusing on the individual and their situation. Ways of doing this (discussed in Chapter 3) include advocacy and voice. The Care Programme Approach (CPA) for people with mental health problems which was introduced in England made some attempt to incorporate these principles in review. The CPA requires Health Authorities, in collaboration with Social Services Departments, to put in place specified arrangements for the care and treatment of mentally ill people in the community. This ensures that people do not become 'lost' in systems. The crucial components of the CPA are:

- an assessment
- a care plan
- a key worker
- regular review

The expectation in the guidelines that review and evaluation should be ongoing and involve the service user reinforces the view that review is an essential part of good practice.

These policy initiatives illustrate the place of review in social work interventions and as an integral part of social work practice that underpins and informs decision making processes. To say that is not to suggest that review is a mechanical process that does not involve social work skills. All review processes involve communication at a number of levels. Workers need to gather information to present to reviews and they have to work with service users, carers and advocates to facilitate their involvement in reviews, assisting them with communication where necessary. The involvement of a number of different professionals as well as services users, carers and advocates indicates the need for negotiation skills.

Requirements of reviews, which consist of overviews, highlight the fourth and perhaps most crucial level of review – that which is part of ongoing work with service users. Best practice requires practitioners to undertake review at every stage of decision making in their work with service users (O'Sullivan, 1999; Bell, 2005). There is sometimes confusion between assessment and review.

Assessment occurs at an early stage in any intervention and may be revisited at different points in the intervention. However, as a stage in a worker's contact with a service user, family or community the assessment process itself is subject to review, both in terms of how the assessment was undertaken and the conclusions that were drawn at the time.

Ongoing reviews are therefore an integral part of good practice. The introduction of care management in adult services led to quite specific requirements for assessment, care, planning, intervention, monitoring and *review* (Orme and Glastonbury, 1993). Similarly, legislation in the area of children and families requires ongoing and regular review. There are also requirements for reviews when specific circumstances require it – such as case conferences to respond to crises, serious case reviews, reviews for reporting processes such as reports to the parole board in criminal justice. Reviews, therefore, punctuate social work, and obviously the end of a social work intervention involves major opportunity for review.

Stages of review

It might seem obvious that social work intervention has a beginning, middle and an end although, as discussions in the next section describe, there have been times when it was assumed that social work intervention would go on indefinitely. Within the stages of social work intervention there are a number of reasons to review situations. Some of these have already been discussed, but a comprehensive list includes:

1. The processes of review are usually embodied in legislation.
2. Some interventions such as task-centred work and solution-focused therapy (see Chapter 8) have review stages built into their methodology.
3. Reviews can provide information about the effects and outcomes of social work intervention; they can contribute to discussions about what is effective and to an evidence base for good practice.
4. Reviews are necessary to monitor the decisions made, the work undertaken and how these relate to the culture.
5. Reviews of actual work undertaken can provide protection for social workers to ensure that their workloads are realistic.
6. Reviews required at agency level for the purposes of demonstrating quality such as *Best Value* and the Care

Standards Act (2000). (See Hafford-Letchfield, 2007, for details of different policies in this area.)

Reasons for review are dictated by the stages in the intervention at which they might occur. These include:

- initial contact and/or referral;
- liaison with others where appropriate;
- decision to allocate, or not, on the basis of initial assessment;
- decisions about methods of intervention on the basis of a more reflective assessment;
- providing services on the basis of assessment and policy criteria;
- identified points at which the situation is appraised (now referred to as care plans): to include further information received from the interventions, the progress being made, and the potential need for a change of approach;
- decisions about ending contact.

Implications of review for practice

While it has been asserted that reviews at all levels have been introduced to try to ensure best practice, there are aspects of review that have had a negative impact. For example DfE (2010) noted the undue importance given to performance indicators and targets which provide only part of the picture of practice, and which have skewed attention to process over the quality and effectiveness of help given.

Reviews associated with 'inspection' are thought to have changed the balance of social work unhelpfully from working with individuals to writing reports or keeping records up to date. Having said that, while social workers often baulk at the time taken to keep records, whether that be manually or on a computer screen, these records can be invaluable not only for providing contemporaneous accounts of events but also documenting the contact that has been made with the family. This can both protect the family by ensuring the service to them can be monitored, and protect the worker by documenting what they have done.

The need for regular review, both internally and externally, to maintain focus on cases recognises that, as a result of workload and other pressures, some cases can take priority over others in practitioners' case loads. Information about workloads helps to account for the work undertaken by any one worker and can be used in workload allocation (Orme, 1995; Baginsky *et al.*, 2010).

While computerised data for the purposes of record keeping is sometimes criticised as not being helpful to the individual's situation (Parton, 2008; Broadhurst *et al.*, 2010) it does have some positive applications. It can lead to greater transparency for service users by flagging up when reviews are required; can provide a record of when reviews are held and what was decided. For workers, computerised records are one way of recording data on tasks undertaken that can be used for the purposes of workloads. Such records can be a rich source of demographic data and area profiles that can identify levels of need but can also build up profiles of areas that can be used in negotiating for resources or initiating social action.

The collection and recording of data about reviews is also a crucial way of ensuring that individuals and agencies are accountable. Reviews, accountability and workload allocation are also key aspects of supervision. Supervision of workers should involve negotiation of the tension between needs and resources. Importantly, it should also enable workers to reflect upon the connections between task and processes in their work (Froggett, 2000). Hence the need to link both, as an underpinning social work process, in this text.

Perhaps the most crucial decision to be made in reflection and review is to end involvement. It is vital that the decision to end contact is justified, to identify what has been learnt about the situation and the intervention and to deal with the service user's and worker's reactions to what has taken place.

Ending interventions

Reflection and review therefore come together in the decision to end intervention. The last stage of reviewing social work intervention comes when the contact ends. Decisions to end intervention depend on a number of factors but underpinning them all is the need for good information. This information can be made available through the presence of a number of different people at the final review stage. However, crucial to an effective review is good written information, including written accounts of the events to date; different perspectives on those events and accurate recording either by ongoing case recording or the completion of computerised forms.

There are, in fact, many endings in social work. Each time we end our contact with users, be it at the end of an interview, home visit or group or community session, important principles of preparing ourselves and the other person for the parting or ending have to be kept in mind. Also social work can be episodic. We can undertake an assessment as social worker, care manager or court officer, and then another worker may be involved. Although for the service user the contact with the agency might not end, the particular relationship between the worker and the user does. Care management and other changes in service delivery mean that more workers will be involved in cases and that contact might be transitory.

Final termination or transfers of work may be planned or unplanned, initiated by service user or worker, mutually agreed or unilaterally decided. Also, increased managerialism, with its focus on targets, response times and throughput means that there is a greater expectation that cases will be closed or passed on to other agencies. Despite this, there is little in the literature on the process of closing cases and ending relationships.

Reasons for closure or transfer to another worker or agency are diverse. They include:

- agreed goals being achieved within a pre-set time;
- service users deciding they want no further contact – either because they have been helped enough, or they are dissatisfied;
- workers leaving or service users moving from the district;
- the end of statutory requirements for involvement (e.g. community supervision of offenders);
- agency policy on time limits for intervention;
- workload management and priority systems;
- resource limitations;
- lack of time and pressure of work;
- advice from supervisor/manager;
- influence of other agencies;
- death of the service user.

In the chapters in the following section on crisis intervention, problem solving and behavioural approaches, we will see how these models were developed to allow for built-in termination. In many of these ending is viewed as a positive step: a way of motivating people by focusing efforts at specified goals. In groupwork, there are ways of anticipating the process of termination systematically, which help understand the possible reactions of denial, backsliding into earlier difficulties, reminiscing and reviewing the worth of the experience (Brown, 1992). Although not all methods of helping or settings for practice lend themselves to a rational model that sets goals, assesses progress and then smoothly starts the process of withdrawing, there are models of good practice.

Increasingly, in arrangements for community care, decisions about closure of establishments or rationalising provision can lead to service users in residential accommodation being relocated geographically. This has implications for relationships with a number of people involved in providing care and support and can cause anxiety. In the case of one establishment for people with mental health problems workers were able to anticipate the closure and relocation of residents by setting up regular meetings to discuss both their fears and their hopes. While this did not totally alleviate the concerns and the disappointments, it did give people, both workers and service users, permission to express their feelings.

Though written some time ago, a couple of articles by Bywaters (1975) help us to understand why so many of our contacts end not with a sense of achievement and neatness but with feelings of loss, work not completed or not even begun. His research into social services revealed bureaucratic, theoretical and psychological drawbacks for service users and workers, which affected both the decision to close or transfer and the process of achieving this. Coupled with the organisational reasons for closing cases, he found that workers often felt they could not control endings and service users were not consulted about the decision. Practitioners often felt that they could do more, or that cases should be left open until a resource such as housing became available. Moreover, feelings of guilt, uncertainty and loss affected the process of handling endings.

In addition, staff experienced ambivalence. They felt guilty knowing that time spent with one person was time not spent with another – therefore closing cases should create more time. They also experienced feelings of loss not because they were 'over-involved' but because they felt uncertainty about their effectiveness. This related to concern about the service user's ability to cope in the future, which impeded a positive approach to endings. Workers felt lost and resentful after putting in a lot of work. These feelings have been exacerbated by managerial decisions to close cases for reasons other than those relating to the wellbeing of the service users and were identified by respondents to Postle's research (2001) who claimed the 'social work side is disappearing'.

Service users and workers may experience transfer or termination of work as a type of crisis (even if the attachment has been short-term) if both have invested a part of themselves. In particular, students on placement report feelings of sadness and anxiety at 'abandoning' those they have worked with. The death of a service user is especially distressing even for those working in specialist services such as palliative care. The principles of reflective practice discussed above are important here because practitioners can experience feelings of bereavement and loss. While at one level they might need reassurance that shedding tears is not unprofessional, they will also need space to explore the impact of each loss. Practitioners are not above theory and are subject to the same emotions as anyone else – what is required is the professionalism to understand the extent and impact of these emotions. Service users and workers may be reminded of earlier losses by the experience of closure. And yet, much in the same way that crisis prevention is possible with 'worry work' and preparation, service users and workers can anticipate endings in advance, enhancing their growth-promoting opportunities.

A good model of ending could incorporate the following:

1. A discussion in the first meeting to establish that contact will not go on for ever. Feelings and perceptions of this are important and need to be handled sensitively. For instance, those in crisis might ask, 'How long will this take?' and, for some, it might be reassuring to know that help will not suddenly be withdrawn. For others, it may be a relief to know that a social worker will not always need to visit.
2. Using the experience of termination or transfer as an opportunity for learning rather than a painful, separating experience. In groupwork, transitions are eased when people are helped to be weaned from the experience – outside relationships and activities are rewarded. Solution-focused and strengths-based perspectives remind us that confirming the individual's self-confidence and self-reliance underlines what he/she has gained and how he/she has dealt with the experience of help coming to an end.
3. Where possible, employing a fixed time limit purposefully, using time itself as a therapeutic agent.
4. Deciding on certain objectives to achieve in the ending phase.
5. Beforehand, exploring a person's feelings about the end of the relationship. This enables both worker and service user

to anticipate possible setbacks, which provide opportunity for worry work. Gradual withdrawal helps, such as reducing the frequency of meetings, arranging for semi-independent living accommodation, progressively leaving longer time with future carers and so on.

6. Introduce the new worker if there is to be one, and talk in the meeting about feelings about the changes. After one social worker did this, the service user vented much resentment but then was free to build a fresh relationship with the incoming practitioner.

7. Help the person construct a helping network in the community, mobilising practical resources if need be. Then carry out a follow-up visit.

8. Explore your own feelings; demonstrate that you will remember the person; have confidence in his or her ability to manage without you but express the goodwill of the agency, whose door is left open should he or she need to return for further help.

9. In some contexts a ritual or ceremonial ending with photographs, a party and a small farewell gift could mark the occasion.

10. Write a closing record, together, if appropriate.

Finally, it is important to remind ourselves that developments are not always linear. Service users can sometimes create situations which might seem to require continued or renewed intervention. It is important to assess each situation carefully – do not dismiss this as attention seeking, but at the same time do not rush to re-establish the former relationship.

Conclusion

Reflection and review are now part of many policy statements but as Bell acknowledges, good reviewing is more than is implied by the formal review mechanisms: 'it explores the process, output and outcomes of social work practice from a range of perspectives' (2005, p. 95). Social workers need to review, reflect on, and to return to, situations that have gone before, in order to make sense of them with new information and new insights gleaned from practice experience, theory and research. Only by reflecting on how we have applied our learning can we ever be sure that we have understood.

While organisation and service user perspectives are important, this chapter has concentrated on the perspective of the practitioner. This is because they are an important agent in the whole process of social work. Practitioners have to implement law and policy, they have to interpret theory and research findings and they have to have open communication with other professionals and service users and carers. They are central to the processes that have been described in this section of the book. Also their interpretations of the situations they meet influence the choice of approaches or methods that they use to work with service users and carers. The next section therefore outlines some of the theory underpinning the major methods of social work intervention.

Practice focus

Michael is a service user in the mental health system, diagnosed with schizophrenia. He has had a rather turbulent history, has no contact with his family and is accommodated in supported housing. Most of the time he has a high degree of independence but because of his lack of family ties he has developed a close relationship with his mental health social worker. As he becomes more independent, he has had to move to accommodation with less staff input. Michael is quite pleased about this but then realises that because the accommodation is in another part of the city he will have to have a change of worker. It is agency policy to allocate cases on a geographical basis.

The social worker tries to help Michael prepare for this. He tells him well in advance of the move and negotiates to continue as the social worker during the transition phase while Michael gets used to his new keyworker. However, as the time for a change of worker gets closer, Michael begins to be more demanding and his symptoms become more acute. The worker likes Michael, has enjoyed working with him and has seen very positive changes in Michael's situation. It would be tempting to try and negotiate with his manager to continue working with Michael. He uses supervision to reflect on all possible motives – both his own and Michael's – for continuing.

At the CPA, all involved help Michael to see what he has achieved. They agree that Michael should contact certain people when he feels sad about losing his former worker. It takes time for Michael to accept his new worker not least because he does not want to get too close in case this worker 'abandons' him too. However, because he has been able to talk about this openly he does not get involved in any of the risk behaviour he has demonstrated in the past.

Point for reflection

This exercise is based on critical incident analysis which has been used in research and training in critical reflection:

Describe a 'critical incident' that has been significant for you in some way in your professional practice. This might be an incident where you think you have made a difference; one which went well; one that was ordinary or typical or one that was demanding. Describe the incident either by writing it down or talking to a fellow student. Explain the context of the incident – that is the detail of the case and the organisation; concentrate on why you think it was 'critical'. Try to identify your thoughts and feelings during and after the incident.

Now read what you have written – or reflect on what you have said to your fellow student. What does this tell you about:

- the kinds of feelings that have been evoked;
- the ideas or theories you were using when thinking about the incident;
- why this incident was 'critical' for you?

Does doing this evoke any other feelings?

Putting it into practice

Identify an event in your practice that involved some kind of review. This might be a Care Plan Assessment, a placement review or a scheduled review of an ongoing case.

- Write down who was involved in the review and in what role: who attended, who chaired?
- Identify what documents were available for the review – were these available to everyone?
- Identify what was the purpose of the review and what was the outcome. How did they relate to each other?
- How was the decision recorded?
- How satisfied do you think the workers were with this process? What makes you think this?
- How satisfied do you think the service users were with the process? What makes you think this?
- What lessons have you learnt from thinking about the review process from the perspective of the people involved? Were you satisfied with the process?

Messages from research

Brandon, M., Dodsworth, J. and Rumball, D. (2005) 'Serious case reviews: learning to use expertise', *Child Abuse Review* (14), pp. 160–76. Findings from research into serious case reviews about the use of expertise (in its widest sense) in the review process.

Further resources

Fook, J. and Gardner, F. (2007) *Practising Critical Reflection: a resource handbook.* Maidenhead, UK: Open University Press. A handbook that describes an approach to critical reflection which demonstrates some skills, strategies and tools which might be used in practice.

Taylor, C. and White, S. (2000) *Practising Reflexivity in Health and Welfare: Making knowledge.* Buckingham: Open University Press. This book is not just for social work but it provides an excellent combination of theory and practice examples to explain the principles behind making knowledge, based on the way workers process and make sense of cases. It provides a useful summary of theories and a glossary.

The Care Programme Association (CPAA) website: http://cpaa.co.uk/ gives information about the Care Programme Approach and information about resources for people with mental health problems involved in this approach.

PART II

Methods of Intervention

The chapters in this section build on the discussion of theory in Chapter 1. Each chapter gives descriptions of how to undertake a particular social work intervention with individuals. The descriptions of the different approaches are accompanied by discussion of the theoretical perspectives on how the method was developed and its effectiveness.

Choosing which interventions to include is problematic because constructions of social work change with different policy initiatives. The ones chosen have been categorised as:

- Counselling
- Crisis
- Problem solving
- Crisis interventions
- Cognitive-behavioural work

However within the different categories the approaches covered are relevant to practice, irrespective of policy changes that have influenced the way that social workers operate. Social work continues to be about relationships, but the relationships that are formed have complex layers. In addition, the work that practitioners undertake within these relationships has a number of different purposes. All social work is about change. Accepting that, the sustaining processes of counselling are evident in work in situations of change involving bereavement loss and crisis. They also give understandings of relationships developed for more focused interventions. Social work is also about problem solving. The range of approaches that focus on problem solving draws on the principles of counselling and working in relationships. These approaches are on a continuum from the strengths-based approaches of solution-focused work through contract making in task-centred work to the more outcomes-focused behavioural approaches.

CHAPTER 6

Counselling

CHAPTER OVERVIEW
- Psychosocial approaches
- Frameworks for understanding psychosocial approaches
- Criticisms of psychosocial approaches
- Counselling in social work: Rogers and Egan
- Incorporating diversity
- Narrative approaches

Context

To state that counselling is fundamental to social work practice is controversial. Criticisms of casework by what has been known as the radical practice movement (Ferguson and Woodward, 2009) have suggested that developments in social work have moved away from a dependence on counselling. Social work has undergone major changes including policy developments such as care management and emerging principles such as user empowerment. Despite these changes, social work still draws on the concepts and skills of counselling (Trevithick, 2005a). The skills, which focus on the relationship, are fundamental to many interventions, even though the context of those interventions may be different. This chapter therefore tries to identify how theories relating to counselling underpin social work.

Developments in social work

Initially, casework meant one-to-one work: working with a case, a situation or a problem. The worker spent time with the person in the situation who was thought to have the problem. Developments involved drawing on theories of human behaviour such as psychosocial development and attachment underpinned by psychodynamic theory.

Hence psychosocial casework developed based on knowledge from psychological sciences: the 'psy' approaches (Healy, 2005; see also Parton and O'Byrne, 2000). It introduced the notion of a 'diagnostic' approach to social work (Richmond, 1922; Hollis, 1964, 1970) which was quite radical in its time as it moved away from the idea of just visiting and supporting people, and suggested social work might bring about change.

Throughout the 1950s and 1960s, Freudian psychoanalytic ideas, particularly personality theory, fed into what became known as psychodynamic casework. 'Psychodynamic' was used because it was based on theory that assumed behaviour comes from movements and interactions in people's minds (Payne, 2005). A criticism of the approach was that workers sometimes relied on the client–worker relationship as an end in itself, spending a lot of time with people which, research suggested, was ineffective (Fischer, 1976). The emphasis therefore turned to intervening to bring about change.

The psychosocial approach as a method of understanding

A psychosocial approach takes into account that people have both inner worlds and outer realities but the way we perceive the world sometimes differs from the way others see it. This is often described as the 'person in-situation' or the 'person in their environment' (the psychosocial). It is the way that the person makes sense of the problem – or just as importantly does not make sense of it – that is the focus of the work. If initial coping strategies or solutions do not seem to alleviate the distress, or in some cases seem to increase anxieties, then it may be worth taking time to explore other explanations.

The psychosocial approach helps to develop a healthy questioning of the obvious. An open mind, imagination and knowledge of personality functioning, human behaviour and emotional suffering are fundamental. This is another way of saying that individuals interact with their environment in unique ways and we have to try to understand underlying feelings and motives that can block people from making optimum use of help.

Many situations in social work cause us to ask what is going on for the person. Understandings based on the psychosocial approach highlight that we should not be too precipitous in dismissing behaviour as just 'difficult', 'non-compliant' or even aggressive. One mantra is: 'think of the opposite'. This does not mean we disbelieve people, but that we should not always accept situations at face value – that is how *we* understand them. We should always try to think of the situation from the perspective of the other person. This is the basis of empathy. So if a woman constantly speaks well of her partner when there are signs that the relationship might be abusive it is important to think about the reasons *why* she needs to believe her own perceptions of her partner. The psychosocial approach is less a system of therapy and more an approach to understanding.

Framework for understanding the psychosocial approach

The theoretical base for psychosocial work is Freudian personality theory, with an emphasis on the ego's capacity for adaptation and problem solving. Basic to the psychosocial approach is knowledge of psychosexual development (see Howe, 1987). According to the psychoanalytic view, the personality consists of three systems: the id, the ego and the superego, which interact dynamically both with each other and with the environment, that is, the individual's living situation (see Milner and O'Byrne, 2002, for an excellent discussion of this). Freud identified *ego-defence mechanisms* which help individuals cope with, among other things, anxiety. Common ego defences are *repression*, whereby painful thoughts and feelings are excluded from awareness; *denial*, where again people 'close their eyes' to threatening actuality but on a more conscious level than repression, and *regression*, where there is a return to behaviour which is immature. In order to assess how realistic and logical the person is in coping with problems and inner conflicts, that is to reveal which method of helping is indicated, elements of personality structure are assessed.

Ego strengths are not a fixed condition but an ever-changing capacity to cope with frustration, control impulses, make mature relationships and use defence mechanisms appropriately. In general, an individual's age, capacity to work through early traumas and the intensity of pressures all affect ego functioning. Many of the situations dealt with in social work can involve challenges to how a person sees her/himself and/or involve loss, of identity, freedom, and so on. In these situations individuals might not desire self-awareness or could not cope with it. Assessing ego strengths assists in understanding how motivated or reluctant the person is likely to be, how much change they can tolerate and what kind of relationship is likely to develop.

Attachment theory

On the basis of Freud's theories, Howe (1995) argues that to understand a person's current performance and competence in social relationships we need to understand the quality of his/her past social relationships. Bowlby (1953) developed a theory of attachment. He argued that to be close to a parent figure, to demand or require comfort, love and attention from that person is a basic desire, just as needing food and warmth are basic desires. These needs lead to what is known as attachment behaviour which includes: proximity seeking; secure base effect and separation protest (Howe, 1995, p. 52). Because Bowlby (1953) originally referred to 'maternal deprivation' debates raged about whether secure attachments could only be provided by biological mothers. This had implications for childcare policy at the time. However Howe (1995) argues that for a human infant to survive and become socially competent it is necessary for him or her to be in close contact with those who are able to provide protection and useful social experiences which is not necessarily the birth mother. When this is not present, the infant can experience loss and separation anxiety which in turn can increase feelings of vulnerability associated with fear and grief which can lead to expressions of pain, anger and depression. These negative experiences and emotions then influence the way the person copes with relationships later in life, especially in times of loss or crisis.

On the other hand, if children have positive experiences of early relationships they learn to handle their own feelings and their reactions to their experiences, which equips them for coping with the complexities of social relationships in adult life. They have self-esteem and feelings of self-worth.

This very brief discussion of attachment theory illustrates how psychosocial approaches in social work emphasise the links between past experiences and current behaviour. In recent years, research has focused on the implications of disorders of attachment in caring arrangements for children (Howe and Fearnley, 2003) but also how the theory has implications for parenting (Howe, 2006) and relationships more generally (Shemmings,

2004). It has also been developed as a form of reflective practice (de Zuluetta, 2010).

Working with relationships

Psychosocial theory, therefore, contributes to our understanding of working with relationships. When helping adults who appear to have 'infantile' needs or, to avoid seemingly pejorative language, whose behaviour is baffling (for example, those who intellectually understand what to do but who do not connect this to their feelings or actions), it might be useful to assess at what stage of psychosexual development they might be stuck or to consider their attachment experiences in early life. When there has been a past trauma, for instance, loss of a parent at a vulnerable age, then, when there is internal or external pressure, some people regress to the stage where these earlier issues were not resolved.

Early studies argued that those clients who seem totally unable to manage their lives, those who antagonise agencies because of their neediness and their inability to care for anyone else can be helped to gradually mature with a worker who feels comfortable in a nurturing relationship. Examples include the patient who is over-concerned with illness but whose numerous tests reveal no abnormality; the person who insists on seeing the social worker at all hours and then is aggressive when limits are imposed. In this context the social worker has been described in a particular role: 'a kind of mother who takes away the mess that the child produces and cleans it up and helps him to do so gradually himself' (Wittenberg, 1970, p. 155).

Creating over-dependence and 'mothering' are unprofessional in social work. Wittenberg's statement means that with some service users workers have to provide understanding, holding and containment. The implications of attachment theory for practice are not about creating dependence within relationships but creating the space to develop healthy relationships.

That said, it should not be assumed that it is always necessary to introduce self-awareness and re-education. Indiscriminate 'laying bare' of feelings can prove overwhelming for some people and interpretation and insight would probably be harmful. The immature ego may need help to increase rather than decrease defences to prevent repressed (unconscious) material from threatening the fragile personality. It is these dangers that highlight the need for social workers to have an understanding of psychosocial methods that can inform decisions about when to refer to trained psychoanalysts.

Psychosocial techniques

Building on Freud's concepts of defence mechanisms, personality structure, transference and counter-transference, resistance and early trauma, Hollis (1970) suggests that the interplay between the 'psycho' and the social aspects lead to clear identification of systems. The focus of work is on:

- *Problems*: which can be intra-psychic, interpersonal or environmental: the 'cause' of a problem, the 'why?' is seen as important.
- *Goals*: which are to understand and change the person, the situation or both; that is, direct and indirect intervention.

To achieve this Hollis identifies two distinct roles:

- The *client's role*: which is somewhat passive, a patient role almost.
- The *worker's role*: which is to study, diagnose and treat the 'person-in-situation' whole.

Treatment processes include establishing a relationship, building ego support via the client's identification with the worker's strengths, helping the client to grow in terms of identity and self-awareness, and working through previously unsettled inner conflicts. A major contribution is obtaining needed practical resources and advocating with others to reduce pressure such that personality change may occur.

Two techniques which follow on from this analysis, sustaining and modifying procedures (Hollis, 1964) have already been described in the Chapter 4.

Criticisms of the psychosocial approach

In the UK, there was concern that social caseworkers would pose as miniature psychoanalysts. Wootton (1959) suggested that rather than search for underlying reasons for behaviour, the social worker would do better to 'look superficially on top'. Other criticisms of the psychosocial approach include:

- It assumed a form of professional omnipotence. For example, whether the worker shared the assessment with the client, depended on the worker's view of the client's ego capacity for self-understanding.
- Clinical and obscure jargon of the psychosocial approach may be offputting.
- It failed to address the broader socio-economic and structural issues that contributed to the problems experienced by clients, or service users.
- There was no acknowledgement of diversity.

Critical sociologists accused social work theorists of favouring the status quo rather than supporting struggle, through collective action, to change society (Healy, 2005). Kenny and Kenny (2000) suggest there is an element of psychic determinism inherent in the tendency to construe cause and effect, often simplistically blaming the past for the present. Hence Ferguson and Woodward (2009) suggest opposition to casework based on a psychosocial approach was not to casework *per se* but to the 'oppressive variants' (Ferguson and Woodward, 2009, p. 22): the failure to connect the individual with their community.

The potential to oppress was because the emphasis was on the person and their psyche, implying that the individual was in some way responsible for her/his problems. In addition, there was an assumption of some kind of 'ideal' way of behaving and being based on an environment which was euro-centric. There was little or no acknowledgement of diversity either of individual lifestyles or the way that different cultures and faiths construct and live in the world.

Notions of a therapeutic relationship, self-disclosure, individualisation and self-awareness, plus the power of the worker to make the diagnosis, have been considered antipathetic to working with diversity. Casework was said to 'pathologise' blackness (Dominelli, 1988) and diverted workers' attention away from systemic racism. The therapeutic techniques of ventilation and reflexive discussion were said to rest on white, middle-class norms regarding the desirability of self-growth and self-awareness (Milner and O'Byrne, 2002, p. 97).

Feminist critiques have suggested early psychosocial approaches also pathologised women, often perceiving the cause of women's problems as being in themselves rather than in their economic and social circumstances (Orme, 2002a). Others point out that the models of human development on which the theories are based can be oppressive to gay, lesbian and bisexual people. The heterosexist bias in theories of psychosocial development is also said to reinforce homophobia (Milner and O'Byrne, 2002).

Healy points out there are continuing attempts to integrate radical and social action with 'psy'chosocial models of intervention (2005, p. 52). To do this, it is necessary to integrate analysis of the structural and cultural injustices that are part of an individual's environment with the individual's reaction to that environment. This integration is the person in their environment. The links between this and the feminist slogan 'the person is the political' are at the heart of attempts that have been made to integrate psychoanalysis with various sociological and political theories including feminist approaches to social work (Orme, 2009).

Some benefits of the psychosocial approach

Kenny and Kenny (2000), while recognising the patriarchal and oppressive potential of psychosocial approaches, also highlight that there is one true constant among all diversity and that is the social worker–client relationship. Echoing constructivist approaches to assessment, they suggest that when clients and workers make sense together, this leads to a shared or empathic understanding (Kenny and Kenny, 2000, p. 33). This sense-making acknowledges that workers need to contemplate ideas such as loss, attachment, individual development, anxiety and transference, and so on, in all interventions. It is commonplace to meet clients who transfer feelings and attitudes on to us that derive from someone else, just as, in counter-transference, we unconsciously respond to the client 'as if' we were that person. For example, clients may relate to us as if we are the all-giving, all-powerful parent they need. If we live up to this fantasy we become unable to say 'no' or to be honest about our limitations.

The strengths of the psychosocial approach are in the emphasis on listening, accepting and avoiding giving direction. The understandings provide a map for directing conversations. For Payne (1997), psychodynamic social work fulfils one of the purposes of social work; it is a method for improving relationships among people within their life situations. This is supported by Trevithick (2005a) who argues that the relationship that practitioners build with service users and carers is central to the social work task, while

Broad (2005) argues that relationship-based practice explores not only the 'how and what' but also the 'why' of practice.

While it is important to understandings in social work, 'classic' psychosocial work is practised less in the UK but has been developed into a number of counselling approaches that draw on the theory and skills. The continuing influence of counselling in social work is related to the centrality of the helping relationship in social work (Healy 2005).

Counselling in social work

Counselling is sometimes used as shorthand for any form of interaction to help people but it is a generic term which covers a number of different schools or approaches. The British Association of Counselling describes counselling and psychotherapy as umbrella terms that cover a range of talking therapies to help people bring about effective change or enhance their wellbeing (British Association for Counselling and Psychotherapy, 2011).

Uses of counselling

Seden (2005) suggests that counselling techniques can be used in many tasks that are undertaken by social workers, including assessment. There are often situations that are difficult to change and people whose behaviour leaves even experienced workers puzzled and floundering. Assessment and intervention in such cases usually cannot be brief and straightforward. Methods are needed to help service users acknowledge their emotional problems and to understand themselves and why they feel powerless to change, or respond to change in unpredictable ways.

Social workers do not necessarily have to undertake in-depth counselling but can refer to other agencies. In a developing 'market' of individuals and organisations that offer counselling, social workers need to have knowledge of, and understand the differences between, various approaches to counselling so that when they refer service users to other agencies, or when commissioning services from these agencies, they are able to make informed judgements about the appropriateness.

Whatever the school of thought or model of counselling followed, generically workers need to be able to listen, observe and respond. As was outlined in the previous chapter, the communication skills needed are attending, specifying, confronting, questioning, reflecting feelings and content, personalising, problem solving and action planning. In order to be effective in active listening and appropriate responses, counsellors must own the following seven qualities:

1. *Empathy or understanding* – the effort to see the world through the other person's eyes.
2. *Respect* – responding in a way that conveys a belief in the other's ability to tackle the problem.
3. *Concreteness or being specific* – so that the counsellee can be enabled to reduce confusion about what he/she means.
4. *Self-knowledge and self-acceptance* – ready to help others with this.
5. *Genuineness* – being real in a relationship.
6. *Congruence* – so that the words we use match our body language.
7. *Immediacy* – dealing with what is going on in the present moment of the counselling session, as a sample of what is going on in someone's everyday life.

The work of Carl Rogers and Gerard Egan is an example of counselling approaches that reflect social work values, such as, accepting the individual, using skills in listening and attending to the information that is given, and working towards joint understanding and decision making about ways forward.

Client-centred counselling

Client-centred (also called person-centred) counselling (Rogers, 1980) is based on the premise that those who seek help are responsible people with power to direct their own lives. It is grounded in the belief that the client is the only natural authority on her or himself. The focus is on the person rather than on solving the presenting problem. Through the counsellor's attitudes of genuine caring, respect and understanding and by demonstrating empathy, congruence and positive regard, people are able to loosen their defences and open themselves to new experiences and revised perceptions (Mearns and Thorne, 1998). As the helping relationship progresses, clients are able to express deeper feelings such as shame, anger and guilt, previously deemed too frightening to incorporate into their sense of self.

During client-centred work the individual moves away from

'oughts' and 'shoulds', that is, living up to the expectations of others. People decide their own standards and independently validate the choices and decisions made. In a climate of acceptance, clients have the opportunity to experience the whole range of their feelings, thereby becoming less defensive about their hidden, negative aspects. They develop 'a way of being'.

This is achieved by a therapeutic relationship that communicates acceptance, respect, understanding and sharing. The counsellor tries to achieve genuineness rather than using depersonalising 'techniques' to create an accepting climate. The counsellor does not have to offer interpretations: staying within the other's frame of reference offers some assurance that clients will not be harmed by this caring approach, which thereby encourages clients to care for themselves.

Egan's systematic helping

Egan's (1981) work provides a framework for the stages or process of the intervention. Each of the stages *exploration, understanding, action* and *evaluation* (shown in Figure 6.1) is represented diagrammatically by four adjacent diamond shapes; these signify the widening and narrowing of focus within each interview, and along the total helping process.

Stage 1: Exploration skills. The worker aims to establish rapport, assisting in the exploration of thoughts, feelings and behaviour relevant to the problem in hand. Asking 'What is the difficulty?' the counsellor tries to build trust and a working alliance, using active listening, reflecting, paraphrasing and summarising skills discussed in Chapter 4. Open questions are used to ascertain which concrete problem the client and the helper need to understand.

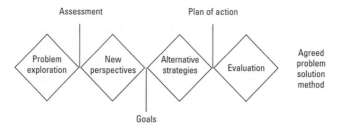

Figure 6.1 Four stages of Egan's model

Stage 2: Understanding skills. The counsellor continues to be facilitative, using Stage 1 skills, and in addition helping the person to piece together the picture that emerges. Themes and patterns may be pointed out to assist in gaining new perspectives, which aid understanding of what the person's goals are, and identifies strengths and resources. The skills lie in offering an alternative frame of reference, using disclosure appropriately, staying in touch with what is happening here-and-now and using confrontation. This latter skill involves encouraging clients to consider what they are doing or not doing, challenging inconsistencies and conflicting ideas in order to tap people's unused resources. Egan views confrontation without support as disastrous, and support without confrontation as anaemic. Hence the timing of confrontation is vital.

Stage 3: Action skills. The worker and the counsellee begin to identify and develop resources for resolving or coping with the causes of concern, based on a thorough understanding of self and situation. The skills lie in setting goals, providing support and resources, teaching problem solving if necessary, agreeing purposes and using decision-making abilities.

Stage 4: Evaluation. An action plan having been chosen and tried, all ideas are reviewed and measured for effectiveness. The counsellor's skills involve active listening together with all those used in previous stages.

If necessary, in a circular fashion, the first stage of wide exploration is resumed as part of the helping process.

In contrast with the Rogerian approach, Egan emphasises the worker's use of influence and expert authority. This makes sense in social work where, in contrast to most counselling, not all clients are willing ones. In adult services with people with mental health problems, in children and families work and in criminal justice social work there are times when we act as agents of control. Social workers use authority that stems from their statutory powers, their position in an organisation, as well as the authority that derives from their knowledge and skill. Although Seden (2005) sees this as a limitation to counselling in statutory social work it can also be an advantage. Authority can be used in counselling to set limits and provide secure boundaries. Equally, practitioners gain authority on occasion from the strength of the relationship and their skills in persuading and negotiating. Although this involves the exercise of power there are ways of sharing power with users by explaining the skills and techniques that are used – and why.

Responses to counselling

There is an irony that while statutory social work becomes more dependent upon approaches that help workers contain situations and operate in the mixed economy of welfare to commission services from other organisations, there is also a growing tendency within society as a whole to turn to counselling. It is argued by some that in the changing organisation of statutory services there is little opportunity to undertake counselling and it has become redundant. Counselling either takes place in specialist settings, such as palliative care (Sheldon, 1997). When it is offered as a specific service it is usually provided by voluntary and independent agencies.

However in childcare practice, there has been a resurgence of interest in psychosocial theories and attachment theory in particular (see Howe, 1995, 1997; DfE, 2011). Often after natural disasters, violent offences, war and other events that involve trauma for groups of people it is reported that teams of counsellors are enlisted to help those involved in the experience (see the next chapter for further discussion). The existence of these teams is testament that, in voluntary sector organisations, and increasingly in the private sector, opportunities for counselling are increasing.

Another argument is that other 'methods' of social work have replaced counselling. However the processes of social work discussed in Part I and many of the methods of intervention discussed in Part II draw upon the principles and skills of counselling. As the section on sustaining and modifying techniques in Chapter 4 illustrates, communicating requires frameworks with which to comprehend the emotional and other meanings vested in the various interchanges. Good practice requires social workers to reflect on the implications of their own and others' actions and reactions. Understandings drawn from these processes inform the decisions of workers about how to intervene.

Incorporating diversity

While good counselling is said to instil confidence in others that they are being accepted and listened to, to avoid being oppressive it must also acknowledge difference. Differences and diversity include age, class, disability, gender, race and sexual orientation, but there are many other aspects of people's experience that might separate them. Counselling relies on empathic understanding of others' experience and frame of reference; this does not mean the experience is shared but that counsellors find ways of understanding the situation from the other perspective.

When the counsellor comes from a different background it might, therefore, be assumed that empathic understanding is not possible. White social workers might be influenced by their own cultural assumptions and fail to recognise the richness of black and ethnic minority cultures. Black workers similarly may feel uncomfortable with white service users, concerned that they will never be able to understand the other's realities.

It is equally problematic to assume that just because both counsellor and service are female, or from the same national or racial background, they will necessarily understand each other. The heterogeneous nature of black and other ethnic minority users of community care services suggests that no one can 'know' everything about them and it would be foolish to assume they did (Stuart, 1996).

If both worker and service user are black, this could create barriers to openness and self-disclosure, especially if the service user believes that the worker has 'sold out' to the establishment, or if the worker over-identifies because of the common bond of racial experience. Equally if both worker and service user are white, the gulf created by class differences can sometimes be ignored

Finally, the very notion of counselling as a model of helping, developed according to Western values, beliefs and perspectives, could be inappropriate to different cultures. For instance, the concepts of self-determination, individualisation, independence and self-disclosure may conflict with values such as interdependence, acceptance and self-control.

The skills of counselling, including careful listening and being open to the views and perspectives of users and carers, are fundamental to avoid stereotyping and making false assumptions about how people make sense of their experiences in the world. This helps to guard against over-simplistic explanations which ignore underlying emotional (and, indeed, structural) factors and cultural differences that contribute to, for example, someone's anger or depression and their ways of dealing with it.

Gender differences

Similar and different issues arise when considering gender differences. Some early feminist literature identified theoretical understandings which, at one and the same time, implies the inferiority of women and provides a key to understanding women's psychology, and their oppression under patriarchy (Eichenbaum and Orbach, 1983; Mitchell, 1984; Chaplin, 1988).

Early feminist social work literature provided some guidelines for working with women arguing that women service users should be seen by female therapists, as only women can understand women. However sometimes gender is not the significant factor, and classic counselling, even when provided by women, does not necessarily espouse feminism. Developments in feminist approaches in social work recognise that assuming that there is an 'essential' femaleness can restrict women's opportunities (Orme, 2002a). In addition, failing to recognise the complexities of women's behaviour might put them, and others, at risk. For example, if it is assumed that women are non-violent, children and older people for whom they care are put at risk (Wise, 1990; Orme, 2002b).

There is vital evidence that, in the initial stages of counselling women who have been beaten, raped or subject to incest, there is a preference for women counsellors. However, in later stages the woman may gain more from a male counsellor who provides a different role model. Such decisions should not be forced on women, but should be arrived at as part of the counselling relationship.

Feminist approaches have also explored the work that has to be done in challenging aspects of masculinity, especially violent behaviour (see Orme, 1995; Cavanagh and Cree, 1996; Day *et al.*, 2009). While it is recognised that having a woman counsellor allows men to develop skills in making positive relationships with women, this has at times been oppressive for women workers. The need for male workers to offer more positive models of masculinity to male clients is just as important (Christie, 2001; Day *et al.*, 2009).

The discussion so far has been based on assumptions based on heterosexual identities. Early psychosocial and counselling work was seen to be imbued with heterosexual assumptions. However Cossis-Brown (2008) points out that the reduced emphasis placed on relationship-based social work has had implications for lesbians and gay men. To work effectively with lesbians and gay men, she argues, requires the ability to work with contradictions. The principles of counselling and using communication skills in relationship-based work are at the heart of good practice that allows people to express their identity.

Older people

Another group for whom counselling is important, but whose needs are sometimes ignored, is older people. Too frequently we assume that problems occur merely because of old age rather than the unique conflicts that face each of us at any age. Ageism makes us fail to see when older people are depressed, abusing alcohol and drugs, having sexual problems, wanting to develop self-awareness or trying to modify behaviour and attitudes (Phillips *et al.*, 2006).

Narrative approaches

Those who have been the exponents of narrative approaches (Parton, 2000; Payne, 2000; Milner, 2001; Milner and O'Byrne, 2002; Fook, 2002) might be surprised to find their ideas discussed in a chapter on counselling. However, there is a clear rationale for dealing with them here. Although focusing more on service users' futures rather than their past, narrative approaches are, it is suggested, another form of counselling. Indeed in some instances the term used is narrative *therapy* (White and Epston, 1990; Payne, 2000). That said, it is important to note that putting narrative approaches with counselling risks recognising only the things that are similar, rather than emphasising differences (Milner, 2001).

Milner and O'Byrne (2002) argue that externalising the internalised story in narrative approaches differs from the insight-giving of psychodynamic approaches. The significant difference is said to be that the focus is not on the person as the problem, but how people become ensnared by problems (Milner and O'Byrne, 2002). However to do this requires looking at the past before going on to the future and involves concepts similar to those in counselling – but reconstructed: *interpretation* is how service users can make meaning of their lives; *resistance* is the way in which service users can resist the influence of problems on their lives (Milner and O'Byrne, 2002, p. 53).

Milner (2001) is clear that narrative approaches, in that they are based on the solution-focused therapy of de Shazer (1988), are future-oriented and therefore relate to the discussions in Chapter 8. It is not necessary to understand the causes of a problem to arrive at its solution. Moreover narrative therapy challenges the belief that a problem defines the identity of people who need help. People should not be thought of *as* problems because they *have* problems.

Narrative approaches are seen to be a necessary and important outcome of the response of social work to postmodernism (Parton and O'Byrne, 2000). As discussed in Chapter 1, this response recognises the oppressive effects of dominant narratives and the ambiguities, contradictions and contingencies of any account of events. It emphasises the need to deconstruct and reconstruct stories with service users. All accounts are perceived to be versions of reality (Fook, 2002) and analysing the narrative is a key factor in how people construct their lives. Importantly, as was said in the discussion of constructivist approaches to assessment in Chapter 2, the purpose is not to get at a single truth, but to get meanings from different perspectives. In deconstructing and reconstructing narratives there are positive ways forward for service users: 'new narratives yield a new vocabulary and construct new meaning, new possibilities and new self agency' (Milner and O'Byrne, 2002, p. 159).

As with all counselling approaches, the role of the worker is vital. The way that he/she asks questions can influence the way narratives are presented. Fook (2002) outlines techniques to aid the reconstruction of the narrative. These include:

- uncovering narratives;
- challenging assumptions that are unhelpful;
- externalising the problem narrative;
- shifting the story to narratives that are enabling and empowering;
- creating an audience. (Fook, 2002, pp. 139–41)

Presenting such a stark outline suggests a rather programmatic approach, but this is not how narrative approaches operate. The significance of the method is not just in the role of the worker but also in the processes of the method. These include:

- externalising the internalised narrative;
- naming the problem;
- discussing the relationship with the problem;
- thickening the plot;
- giving narrative feedback. (Milner and O'Byrne, 2002)

Hence while the emphasis is very different – concentrating on the discourse (what is said) rather than the person – narrative approaches offer opportunities to understand people's interpretation of both the internal and external world. Also, in that they offer a relationship over time and are based on respect for the person, they do incorporate some aspects of counselling. As Parton and O'Byrne comment in their introduction to what they see as a new social work practice:

> It may be that the psychodynamic approach's greatest contribution had little to do with providing an understanding of the functioning of the ego, the super ego and the id but the importance of the validation that a person receives simply in telling their story to an attentive listener. (Parton and O'Byrne, 2000, p. 12)

Conclusion

This chapter leads the section on interventions because, both chronologically and in terms of the importance of the theories outlined, it is fundamental to all social work interventions. In focusing on the need to find explanations for the way people feel, the way they behave and indeed the way they feel about the way they behave, psychosocial approaches enable social workers to begin to explore the interrelationship between the individual and the environment. Admittedly this was initially a very narrow view, and the focus on the individual meant that service users, or clients, tended to be pathologised: the problem was seen to rest in them. However in moving away from the pathologising tendencies it is vital that social work does not abandon the individual totally. Even proponents of radical social work recognise the centrality of the relationship in good social work practice: what they do not accept is the social worker as therapeutic 'expert' (Ferguson and Woodward, 2009).

As the rest of the book will illustrate, whether social workers are working with individuals, groups, families or communities it is important to try to discern how the individual makes sense of his/her experiences and to work with their strengths. This is not to deny that political and socio-economic forces, together with the organisation of social work agencies, are powerful influences in the way that social problems, and those who experience them, are constructed. However to ensure that we work in a non-oppressive way we need to ensure that we do not make assumptions about how people experience their world but try to find ways of enabling them to express exactly who they are and what they make of their experiences.

Practice focus

Mrs Todd is a woman in her 70s suffering from cancer. She has no immediate family and lives alone. After the death of her husband, some twenty years ago, Mrs Todd lived an active life. She was employed as an administrator and was financially secure so was able to travel, join organisations and make new friends. She had also given a great deal of support throughout her life to her parents until their deaths.

In recent years Mrs Todd has lost contact with her friends, ceased all her activities and is now quite lonely. Her physical symptoms are being managed by medication, and she attends a centre one day a week. However she is depressed and finds it difficult both physically and emotionally to do very much for herself. While the staff at the centre realise her mood might be related to her medication, they are also aware that her illness has an impact on her sense of self. She has moved from being an active, independent professional woman to one who can no longer manage. Having been house proud and able to manage shopping online and other ways of maintaining her independence, she is now finding it all too difficult and she is distressed that 'things are falling apart'.

During sessions with a counsellor from the palliative care team it emerged that despite having had many positive life experiences Mrs Todd had desperately wanted to be looked after. Now that she needed looking after she felt ambivalent. She felt that asking for help meant being a 'failure'. The counsellor was able to encourage Mrs Todd recognise that we all need looking after at some time and the messages she was carrying from her childhood, while they had helped during other crises in her life were not necessarily relevant at this point. Gradually Mrs Todd was able to accept some help in the home. This made it more comfortable and she was able to ask neighbours to visit and they offered practical help.

Putting it into practice

Practising counselling is difficult. As has been said, putting counselling theory into practice usually involves feedback through supervision, often using video links or special interviewing rooms. However there are things that can be done to make us more aware of some of the processes that take place in the helping relationship. The practice of writing a process recording is very useful and combines both the use of counselling in practice and the exercise of reflecting on that practice.

In a process recording the worker/student writes a very detailed account of what happens in an interview interaction. It is important to choose an interview that, for whatever reason, was significant for you. Also when choosing an interview, focus on only a part of it, otherwise the account will be too long and/or too superficial. Again, choose the part that was significant to you, whatever the reason.

1 Write down everything that happens in the part of the interview that you are focusing on: who said what, the words that are used, the silences, the non-verbal signals – everything you can remember about your own interventions and those of the service user (and anyone else who might have been involved).
2 Now re-read the account and write down what you think was going on for the service user, bearing in mind some of the ideas and theories that have been discussed in this chapter. What do the words used mean? What story is the person telling? How is the person reacting to you? Is he or she relating to you in ways that are unexpected? Why might this be so?
3 Now read the account again and write down what was happening for you in the interview/interaction. Why have you chosen this section of this interview? How did you react to the situation? How did you react to the things that were said? Why do you think you reacted in that way? What made you decide to do the things that you did/said?
4 Now read all three accounts to see if you can relate what is recorded (and what happened) to the theories that have been discussed in this chapter.

Messages from research

Broad, G. (2005) 'Relationship-based practice and reflective practice: holistic approaches to contemporary child care social work', *Child and Family Social Work*, 10, pp. 111–23. This article gives a useful overview of the literature on psychosocial and 'relationship-based' practice drawing on her research with practitioners to describe how good practice requires a good relationship, which itself depends on good practice.

Shemmings, D. (2004) 'Researching relationships from an attachment perspective: the use of behavioural, interview, self-report and projective measures', *Journal of Social Work Practice*, 18(3), pp. 299–314. This article provides important insight into how practice can be researched and includes some illustrative examples using practice-related material.

Further resources

Cossis-Brown, H. (2002) 'Counselling', in Adams, R., Dominelli, L. and Payne, M. (eds) *Social Work: themes, issues and critical debates.* Basingstoke: Palgrave Macmillan.
An introductory chapter that gives an overview of counselling and its place in social work.

Seden, J. (2005) *Counselling Skills in Social Work Practice.* Buckingham: Open University Press.
This text discusses the basic principles and practices of counselling and their implications for social work practice.

The Psychosocial Working Group (PWG) was established in 2000 as a collaboration between academic institutions and humanitarian agencies committed to the development of knowledge and best practice in the field of psychosocial interventions in complex emergencies. It includes the *Psychosocial practitioners network* – the aim of which is to work with key practitioner, academic and policy agencies to set up a web-based network to create an opportunity for dialogue between practitioners, academics and policy makers. The website is at: http://www.forcedmigration.org/psychosocial/PWGinfo.htm.

Crisis interventions

Introduction

Individuals who come to social work agencies are frequently in crisis precipitated by homelessness, debt, difficulties with looking after children, the onset of dementia or other aspects of living. Others may have experienced or are experiencing trauma and loss. This loss may be an actual one, for example as a result of bereavement, divorce or illness. However, many of the circumstances which constitute crises also involve loss: loss of a home or a job; loss of life as we know it because of illness, injury, mental ill health and many other life events. Some crises are developmental: part of the experiences of the life cycle. Other crises are acute events that have affected the capacity of the person to function. For some people, crises might seem to be a permanent way of living, and they develop mechanisms for coping. For others, one seemingly small event might precipitate feelings of helplessness and render the person incapable of acting. Because people react differently it is therefore important for social workers to understand what is meant by 'crisis' as it relates to social work intervention.

People who come to social work in crises want the immediate problem solved and problem solving work focusing on solutions is therefore important, as explored in the next chapter. However the theories explored in the previous chapter indicate that, while social workers should focus on resolving the immediate issues, understanding of what has caused them and what influences how the person is coping can be complicated but equally important. As

Healy (2005) points out, crisis intervention is a form of problem solving practice based on psychiatry while task-centred approaches draw on theories from cognitive and behavioural psychotherapies. This leads to some important distinctions between the two approaches.

Situations that involve change, no matter how much that change is welcomed, usually involve losing something, giving up something. Therefore one of the basic functions of social work is working with people facing loss and change. For this reason, the theories of bereavement are also explored in this chapter as they are also relevant to understanding reactions to crises.

What do we mean by 'crisis'?

Because social work interventions are frequently undertaken with people in crisis, the word is generally misunderstood and used in something of a dragnet fashion, describing a variety of problems, needs, stresses and emergency states. Teams talk about crises when they mean that an urgent referral has come in or that they can only 'do crisis work', that is, engage in minimal activity because of overwork. This signifies a lack of understanding of the concept of crisis and methods of intervention. Discussions in this chapter aim to help practitioners avoid uncritical and undifferentiated use of the concept and to apply and develop the processes associated with what is called crisis intervention or crisis work.

Defining crisis is difficult (O'Hagan, 1986) and hampered by the layperson's portrayal of crisis as a drama, panic, chaos and so on. The first study of the ways in which individuals reacted to psychologically hazardous situations formulated the concept of crisis (Caplan, 1964; Lindemann, 1965). Rapoport further defined a crisis as 'an upset in a steady state' (Rapoport, 1970, p. 276).

This led to explorations of how a sense of loss associated with unexpected, accidental or developmental life transitions throws an individual into a state of helplessness, where coping strategies are no longer successful in overcoming problems and where the person's psychological defences are weakened. Crises are not necessarily unusual or tragic events; they can form a normal part of our development and maturation. While the steady state (also called 'homeostasis' or 'equilibrium') is usually maintained by human beings through a series of adaptations and problem solving processes, crises require more. What happens in a crisis is that our habitual strengths and ways of coping do not work; we fail to adjust because the situation is new to us, or it has not been anticipated, or a series of events become too overwhelming. New solutions are usually needed to manage the hazardous event that has precipitated feelings of disequilibrium.

If a human being is overpowered by external, interpersonal or intrapsychic forces (in other words, conflicting needs) then harmony is lost for a time. One important thing to remember is that crises are self-limiting; they also have a beginning, middle and end. Caplan (1964) postulated that the crisis period lasts for up to six weeks. In the initial phase there is a rise in tension as a reaction to the impact of stress; during this time habitual ways of trying to solve problems are called on. If first efforts fail, this causes tension to rise even further, as the person gets upset at his/her ineffectiveness (the middle phase). This state of mind results in the final phase, when either the problem is solved or the individual, needing to rid him/herself of the problem, redefines it for instance as something less threatening; or, alternatively, the problem is avoided altogether, for example by distancing oneself from it. (The same phenomenon of protest, despair and detachment is familiar to workers who understand the application of attachment theory to separation traumas of young children.) It can be seen that crises have a peak or turning point; as this peak approaches, tension mounts and energy for coping is mobilised – we 'rise to the occasion' (Parad and Caplan, 1965, p. 57).

While the notion of a neat progression through the stages is sometimes questioned, it is generally accepted that, during the disorganised recovery stage, people are more receptive to being helped because they are less defensive and need to restore the predictability of their worlds; we all seek some kind of balance in our daily lives. That said, there are some families and individuals who seem to thrive on living in a constant state of crisis; they lurch from one seemingly appalling state of chaos to another, on the precipice of eviction, fuel disconnection, abandonment and despair. This chronic state may be part of the lifestyle and should not to be confused with concepts of acute crisis discussed so far.

Crises can be perceived as a threat, a loss or a challenge. The threat can be to one's self-esteem or to one's sense of trust. The loss might be an actual one or may be an inner feeling of emptiness and isolation. When viewed as a challenge, a crisis can encompass not only danger but also an opportunity for growth. This is especially so when new methods of solving problems are found or when the person finds that he/she can cope. Similarly, because crises can revive old, unresolved issues from the past, they can add to the sense of being overwhelmed and overburdened (a double dose); at the same time, however, they can offer a second chance to correct non-adjustment to a past event. Increased mental energy often accompanies the vulnerability and, when it is no longer being used to repress ill-resolved old problems, can be used to develop coping mechanisms.

Practice focus

The ward sister of a nearby hospital contacted the hospital social worker who had spent some months working with the Smith family during the period of hospitalisation of their nine-year-old daughter, Sophie, who had become disabled following a road accident.

The Smiths had been thought to cope well at the time of the accident, itself a crisis. They had worked with the social worker planning for Sophie's return home and adaptations and equipment were installed in the home. However, when the ward sister gave the Smith's the actual discharge date Mr Smith had become uncontrollably tearful, denying that Sophie was ready to come home and saying that he could not cope. The social worker identified this as part of the period of crisis. She spent time with Mr Smith focusing on his concerns and how he and his wife had coped to date reassuring him that his emotions were normal and that all the resources would be made available.

The specificity of a discharge date had triggered off inner conflicts in Mr Smith, only partially resolved and he expressed concerns that the stress of coping might cause his wife to leave him. It emerged that she had done so some years before. Rather than seek help with their unhappy marriage, the couple had resigned themselves to their disappointment in each other, never talking about the past and trying to pretend that their problems had never existed. Their efforts and emotions had then been focused on their daughter. In order to uncouple the symbolic links between past and present needs and fears, the worker focused in the short term on how they had coped in previous periods of difficulty or crisis.

In the long term following the short-term crisis intervention, the worker discussed with the Smiths the possibility of accessing more open-ended marital counselling.

The immediate problems caused by Mr Smith's reactions to his daughter's discharge had to be dealt with but it was apparent that this was not a situation where all problems could be resolved quickly. Mr Smith's reactions indicated that there were underlying issues other than practical problems to be dealt with. While the social worker might have been under pressure from the hospital to ensure that the bed was vacated a 'fire-fighting' response was not appropriate. The Smiths perceived themselves as having no autonomy or command over their problems, tension had mounted and Mr Smith's thinking in particular had become disintegrated so that little mental energy was left over to use inner and outer resources. This obviously put pressure on the relationship. Without help, either of the Smiths could deteriorate into a major state of personality and behavioural pathology – a marital breakdown or what is commonly termed a 'nervous breakdown' could have occurred. This would not be helpful for them or for Sophie: further problems would have been caused if the family situation had broken down. This illustrates how sometimes just dealing with the practical or immediate problems is not always enough.

Having said that, Thompson (1991) criticised what he calls pure crisis 'theory' because it can be dissociated from structural factors of oppression and relies on clinical terms that can pathologise the individual experiencing trauma. Caring for Sophie might involve real financial problems and precipitate other demands on Mr Smith in terms of the time he would need to devote to the care of his daughter while in full-time work. In addition, his reactions might have been exacerbated by having to cope with his daughter's accident according to societal expectations of male behaviour that he should 'cope' without showing emotions. Such factors have to be considered as part of the overall assessment.

Crisis and stress

Occasionally, the word 'stress' is used interchangeably with crisis. However, the concept of stress tends to evoke only negative connotations, for instance, that stress is a burden or a load under which people can crack. In comparison, we have seen that the state of crisis need not have this harmful outcome. Crises occur throughout life, they are not illnesses; we constantly make adaptive manoeuvres in order to cope and maintain our steady state. If we meet a novel situation, experience too many life events, or become overloaded with old, unresolved conflicts, then a crisis occurs. This is a time-limited process during which we become disorganised in thinking and behaving. Mounting tension can result in the generation of mental energy for getting the problem solved. On a positive note, the outcome can include improved mental health, when new methods of coping are found or when there is a second chance to tackle an earlier hazardous event. It should be remembered that the outcome of the crisis can depend, not just on skilled intervention, but also on the quality of the person's social support network (Parry, 1990).

Crisis therefore contains a growth-promoting possibility; it can be a catalyst, raising the level of mental health by changing old habits of problem solving and evolving new ways of coping. In addition, the concept of stress carries within it a sense of longer-term pressures, which may largely derive from external pressure as opposed to internal conflict. Crisis, on the other hand, appears as a short-term phenomenon where the individual rapidly tries to re-establish previous harmony. Earlier levels of functioning may have been inadequate, but that is where the person's perception of equanimity lies: where crisis resolution is less than optimum, lower levels of coping may result.

There is a relationship between life events and stress. A state of crisis can occur as a result of stress when making social readjustments such as moving house, having a first child or becoming unemployed. What is important is that what constitutes unbearable stress for one person may not be so for another. Students are always surprised when they compare their views of stressful events with their colleagues; some dread Christmas, others lose their sense of coping when faced with academic work. Thus, it is the meaning that people attach to these 'uneventful' events that matters – maybe someone links Christmas symbolically to an unsatisfactory time in the past, or someone whose self-esteem was bound up with academic success attaches great significance to results. The same is true for service users – what the event means to them is what matters, not whether we think it is serious or not.

Framework for understanding crisis intervention

The differences between stress and crisis reflect some of the important factors that underpin a framework for understanding crisis intervention. These include:

1. *Theories* and important concepts, which contribute to the identification of crisis. In the main these theories are developed from the 'psy' disciplines discussed in the previous chapter.

    (a) Psychoanalytic theories of personality (see Chapter 6) where the ego directs energy for problem solving, appraises reality and helps us to cope, adapt and master conflicts.

    (b) Erikson (1965), building on ego psychology, suggests that we grow by managing psychosocial crisis points, which are transitional points in our life cycle towards maturity.

    (c) Learning theory contributes in relation to ideas about cognitive perception; role modelling and repetitive rehearsal of effective problem solving (see Chapter 9).

    (d) These contributions fuse with those from research into grief reactions (Lindemann, 1965) discussed below and those of time-limited, task-focused work dealt with in the following chapter.

2. *Problems* for which this approach is applicable may not even seem like problems. They can be changes, such as becoming a teenager, as well as situational or unanticipated crises, such as promotion or illness. Furthermore, as we have seen, crises can occur at any time when a person perceives a threat to his/her life goals. It is the meaning of the event to the unique individual that matters. Problems are usually current and pressing ones; routine early history taking would be inappropriate. So too would organisational arrangements such as waiting lists or long-drawn-out allocation procedures. Chronic crisis situations cannot be dealt with by this approach alone – longer-term, in-depth work is often necessary.

3. *Goals* are kept to a minimum. They include relief of current life stressors, restoration to the previous level of coping, learning to understand what precipitated the condition, planning what the person can do to maintain maximum autonomy and contact with reality, and finding out what other resources could be used. When current stresses have their origins in past life experiences, the goal might be to help the person to come to terms with earlier losses to reduce the risk of future vulnerability.

4. *The client's role* is to review and question the hazardous event in order to understand how the state of crisis occurred. At times, people take unwise decisions or make inappropriate suggestions for solving the problem, so the worker takes advantage of the person's lowered defences and willingness to take advice, thereby inhibiting flight, for example premature plans for the future. Indeed, a lot of the work for clients is to

remember that there is a future: by 'telling the story to themselves' cognitive awareness is improved. Sharing the experience and the feelings with family or others in the support network strengthens these resources which, in their distress, some clients forget are there. Disintegration is also prevented when the client assumes responsibility for some small practical task.

5. *The worker's role* is to give information and advice, to be active, directive and systematic, if need be. It is essential to be authentic as part of the promotion of reality testing and adjustment. Setting time limits, for example four to six contacts, encourages the person to face up to the future without fear or shame that he/she will never be independent again. While cognitive restructuring and release of tension are the aims of this approach, self-understanding as discussed in the previous chapter need not be part of the worker's plan for the client. Teaching how to split problems into manageable pieces and acting as a role model for effective problem solving in the acute stage is more helpful. To do this, workers must put themselves into a position of 'standing still', that is, remaining calm and being able to 'bear it' when confronted with someone in crisis. The danger in crisis intervention is that the caregivers, surrounded by people who want something done can go into crisis themselves, not thinking clearly about what needs to be done.

Techniques of crisis intervention

Techniques for intervening in crisis situations provide help in the initial, ongoing and final stages. In the first interview it is essential that the focus be kept on the present circumstances of the crisis event. Asking 'What happened?' thereby encourages the person's cognitive grasp of the situation. Comments such as 'You must feel awful' or 'No wonder you are upset' help to draw out the affective responses (that is, feelings) which block thinking. The worker and client together try to make an assessment of the actual event and the causes that seem to have triggered it. It is necessary to gauge what ego strengths (see previous chapter) someone has so that his/her normal coping resources can be gleaned. Often asking how the person has reacted in other, similar, situations can do this.

Having gained some idea of available and potential resources, the worker outlines the next step, asking 'What is the most pressing problem?' or 'What is bothering you most?' The client is then asked to settle on one target area, the worker confirming this by saying 'So the most important thing is …?' Obviously, these are not formulae for copying, they are suggestions as to what to cover in the initial period of disorganisation when the worker conveys hope, shows commitment to persevering while cutting the overwhelming problem down into manageable bits (known as partialising the problem). A contract for further work is spelled out in specific, concrete terms such as 'Let's concentrate on … You do … I'll do …' These are not problem solving contracts such as those used in task-centred work, but help give the person some agency, some influence and/or control over what seems an uncontrollable situation. Realistic optimism is used to reduce the client's anxiety and perception of hopelessness, concreteness helps to keep the person in touch with reality. The aim at this early stage is to start to build a relationship based not on time but on the worker's expertise and authenticity to restore the client's sense of trust. Because of this, it might be necessary to have a number of short meetings at regular intervals (even daily). This may appear to create a sense of dependence, but the worker should always be clear that this is just an interim period.

As the client's thinking is clarified, it is necessary to re-establish a sense of autonomy, by giving him/her something to do before the next meeting. This can be achieved, for instance with someone frozen into inaction, by getting him/her to say when next you need to meet again. In any event, letting individuals decide on the schedule for help such as 'I think I need to see you four more times over the next two weeks' builds self-reliance into the agreement and prevents undue dependence in the longer term.

Further contact in the middle phase sees the worker centring on obtaining missing data, for example, 'Can you tell me more about …?' Although the emphasis is still on the here-and-now there may be links with past conflicts not recognised in the earlier phase of staying with the presenting issues. Pointing out possible connections helps the person to correct cognitive perception while keeping the problem, rather than fantasy or distortion, in the foreground. In addition, one way of helping people keep a perspective is to recognise that he/she has had past crises and has coped with these. Discussing those coping mechanisms sometimes gives good indications about what approaches might work in the current situation. The helper has to help show the difference between 'what is' (real) and 'If only'. Maybe Mr Smith would have wished his daughter had not had the accident. But it is not possible to reverse this and plans had to be made to assist her and others to live with her disability.

Letting the person talk helps to relieve tension; ventilating feelings can release mental energy for tackling past worries. Help is given to sort out what worked and did not work in attempting to solve the problems; 'So you did ... Did it work?' Alternative solutions are weighed; exploring overlooked resources assists in restoring equilibrium and also develops a pattern (that is, new habits) in being able to use such help in the future. By sorting out specific tasks together, aiming for achievable goals, the social worker acts as a role model for competent problem solving; for instance, setting homework, 'Before we next meet I'd like you to think how you could ...', sets the stage for encouraging a change in thinking, feeling and action.

The termination phase of crisis intervention should have been built into the original agreement. Once the state of crisis is overcome and homeostasis restored it would be harmful to prolong this type of approach as it could ignore the natural growth potential present in all human beings. Reminding the client how much time there is left; reviewing progress and planning for the future prevent dependency (that is, lowered functioning). However, premature termination, 'I can cope now, so I don't want to see you any more', could be a 'flight into health' (Rapoport, 1970) not a well thought-through decision.

Crisis and diversity

Although the underpinning theory might help to guide interventions it is always important to remember that the crisis has to be understood from the perspective of the person experiencing it and this might be influenced by their race, gender, age and other differences between people. When differences are not understood or are misconstrued this can have disastrous consequences.

For example, where the situation involves someone whose cultural norms involve different ways of reacting to stress assumptions about what is 'normal' can lead to misinterpretations of the reactions as mental ill health. The very experience of not being accepted and understood can lead to crises. In the 1990s, Aros-Atolagbe (1990) found that second-generation black people in the

UK suffered tremendous crises of cultural identification; alienation produces more stress, which may precipitate a temporary breakdown.

Individuals and ethnic groups obviously vary in their reactions but many immigrants may go through a pattern of adaptation to an unfamiliar, and probably discriminating, environment. Asylum seekers and others who face oppression when they enter the country may react in similar ways. The loss of support networks together with a sense of powerlessness means that the process of emigrating goes through critical phases such as: excitement, disenchantment, perception of discrimination, identification crisis, and marginal acceptance. Such feelings are exacerbated when the reasons for leaving the homeland have been traumatic, for example refugees from war-torn countries.

In the case of asylum seekers the situation arises more immediately. Levels of stress caused by the sense of dislocation can exacerbate a state of crisis when this stress is either ignored or denied. Excitement might be more a sense of hope, which often turns to despair when officials who deal with applications take no account of these experiences or emotions.

Explanations for the misdiagnosis of people from different cultural backgrounds include the misinterpretation by workers of reactions to crisis and loss. On the one hand, some groups may be able to express their reactions by overt demonstrations of emotion. In some cultures holding a wake or similar event to allow the outward expression of personal grief is the norm, while in the UK, open displays of emotion, although becoming more acceptable, are still frowned upon in some generations. On the other hand, cultural expectations of what has to be tolerated without comment or expression of emotion may be interpreted as depression by workers who expect clients to be prepared to 'talk through' situations (Hong Chui and Ford, 2000).

Similar misinterpretations may occur on the basis of gender, where stereotypical assumptions lead workers to expect that men and women cope with difficult situations in different ways. The social worker in the case of Mr Smith, for example, was able to accept that his uncontrollable tears were a perfectly normal reaction to the events with which he had to cope. This is an important message in a culture that has deterred men from using tears as an appropriate means of stress relief.

Therefore, we can see that the signs of someone in crisis actually might be difficult to spot, or the behaviour may be open to different interpretations. However, like grief, some of the responses follow a typical or classical pathway and this can give us some clues. We know that in the period of distress the person is striving to gain control, and is open to suggestions which will aid recovery: phrases may include 'I can't cope', 'I feel a failure', 'I don't know where to turn' or 'It is hopeless'. Often thoughts and behaviour are agitated, confused, hostile, ashamed or helpless. People may become irritable or withdrawn from their friends and relatives. Attempts to solve difficulties seem chaotic and unfocused. Other signs may be physiological, so that complaints about sleeplessness, tension and headaches (see Parry, 1990) may be mentioned by someone in crisis.

A more contentious debate in the context of diversity is that taking place in relation to disability as loss and therefore a crisis. The 'tragedy' model of disability that is based on disability as being the 'loss' of normality has been criticised by the disability movement. It is associated with the tendency of social workers to individualise problems and to see the person as impaired as opposed to the environment as disabling. However concern has been expressed that denial of feelings of loss experienced by those with an illness and/or disability could lead to people with disabilities being unable to express their negative feelings about their impairment. Approaches to loss and grief which emphasise that it is the individual's construction of their situation that is important might help resolve differences in these approaches (Sapey, 2004).

Bereavement and loss

Throughout this chapter we have made reference to the fact that crises are not necessarily dramatic or unusual events. Different life events and the reactions they precipitate are sometimes called developmental crises because they are associated with loss. An example of such a developmental crisis is childbirth. This is a biological event and usually associated with gains. However, the birth of a child precipitates many changes for women, some of which involve loss. For women who are giving up work there is loss of economic independence and loss of the social environment of the work place. For women who plan to return to work, there are other losses to face; loss of independence and freedom and, if in a relationship, the loss of intimacy. Similar and different losses may be experienced by men who become fathers. No matter how 'planned' the pregnancy is, all these things can create crises because of the potential for unexpected emotional reactions to the various losses.

It is the concept of loss, present in many crisis situations, that makes bereavement theory so important for helping understand crises and anticipating reactions to some of the developmental crises (such as birth, adolescence, ageing/retirement and, of course, death). Other situations, often more difficult to anticipate, similarly involve loss and therefore the sense of being bereaved. These include divorce, separation from children or partners, disability by either accident or disease and the impact of illness such as dementia, stroke or multiple sclerosis. Situations, such as loss of employment, housing and freedom can precipitate many practical problems, but sometimes the capacity to deal with those is affected by the emotional response to the actual loss, and the loss of identity or self of sense that comes with it. Workers therefore have to be prepared to deal with the range and complexity of emotions associated with loss and bereavement in all aspects of their work.

One of the earliest texts to discuss the physical and emotional effects of grief and bereavement identified five stages of typical reactions to grief (Parkes, 1986). Listing these is not intended to provide a formula for how to chart people's progress through them. They are an aid to understanding people's reactions to loss, and provide a basis for formulating the kinds of intervention that are empathic and facilitative to people in crisis.

The stages are:

- alarm
- searching
- mitigation
- anger and guilt
- gaining a new identity

In each of these stages physical and emotional changes occur, which are associated with coming to terms with the loss, with the separation from the person who has died, or left. Symptoms occur which are physical, such as disturbance of appetite and/or sleep, palpitations and breathlessness. Behaviour is displayed which may seem bizarre or morbid, such as searching for the person, denying his/her death and continuing to live life as if he/she was still present. Emotions expressed can be extreme and include anger with self, the deceased person and professionals who may be held responsible for the loss, guilt at not being able to prevent the loss, or at feelings and behaviour just prior to the death. These can be painful and powerful.

The importance of identifying the range of experiences associated with grief and bereavement (Pincus, 1976) is that workers can accept the bereaved person with all his/her ambivalences, contradictions and complexities. In accepting and understanding the stages of grief work, they can give reassurance that while each grief experienced is personal and unique, the person experiencing it is not abnormal in the ways that he/she expresses it. Having said that, there are occasions when people, for a variety of reasons, become fixed in a particular grief reaction or display extremes of behaviour. In these circumstances having a framework to help assess an individual's coping strategies and to identify particular ways of working with these to develop and strengthen the person's own resources is helpful. Knowing when to stay with a person and listen, when to offer practical tasks and when to introduce them to a support group, or to more specialised help, is part of understanding the stages of grief and bereavement.

However the 'stages' of grief approach has been criticised for being too programmatic and too rooted in attachment theory. It ignores the fact that the way that an individual constructs death emanates from his/her particular values and attitudes (Payne, 2005) and behaviour can be influenced by differences in, for example, race and gender. Silverman describing mourning as the psychological process by which an individual adapts to the loss of a loved one emphasises 'the social process including the cultural traditions and rituals that guide behaviour after a death' (Silverman, 2004, p. 226).

Another criticism is that the final stage, 'gaining a new identity', suggests that individuals are encouraged to 'move on' and 'get over' bereavement by becoming detached from the person they have lost. It may be that the new identity is more to do with having to cope with life without the presence of the other person. The bereaved person has to relocate him/herself in the world. This has led to recognition that work might include a 'dual process model' of coping with bereavement (Currer, 2002). This acknowledges both the stress of the loss and the changes that result from it which leads to a dual focus for the work – loss and orientation. Most people require both, but Currer (2002) suggests that social workers working with a 'staged' model might be more focused on restoration, helping people with practical changes and adjustments, and opportunities to focus on loss might be missed.

However as Silverman (2004) points out people have to cope with both extreme feelings caused by the loss but also with changed social context: another type of relationship has to be constructed with the deceased. Because of this, she suggests that mourning does not end, there is a constant adaptation to, and accommodation of, change:

> More than a life is lost. A relationship is also lost. A self in that relationship is lost and a way of living and relating to life is lost, as well. (Silverman, 2004, p. 228)

Of course the impact of the loss will relate to the nature of the relationship and will be influenced by the ego strengths discussed in the previous chapter, including experiences of attachment. For some where there are positive attachments, feelings of anger can accompany feelings of sadness – anger at being abandoned. In less positive relationships, the feelings of anger might be paramount – anger that differences and difficulties were not resolved.

Grief is therefore a period of transition and Currer (2002) suggests that oscillation (moving between the states) is the key to adaptive behaviour. This has to involve both assimilation and accommodation of the new situation (Silverman, 2004), but this does not constitute recovering or 'getting over' the lost person. To aid adaptation Silverman (2004) identifies that at the point of immediate loss, it is important for the bereaved person to be helped to give 'witness' to the relationship. This requires workers to:

- recognise the need to grieve
- give accompaniment to the grieving person
- give support in relation to re-engagement

According to Silverman (2004) transition takes place on several levels and in no particular order. Therefore, the notion of being 'fixed' at a particular stage might not be helpful. In addition, throughout any support that is given, workers should always recognise that there may be a future need to grieve. Nevertheless, the 'stages' of the process are still a means of understanding the swings in emotion, and the sometimes unexpected emotions experienced in grief work. This approach was seen as helpful by Sapey (2004) in his discussions about experiences of loss felt by people with disabilities.

Coping with catastrophe

Grief is often seen as a personal and individual experience but in recent years it has manifested itself differently. The practice example at the end of the chapter illustrates a grief reaction now known as post-traumatic stress disorder. This phenomenon can occur as a reaction to significant loss, not just loss of life. Nuttman-Shwartz and colleagues (2010) for example describe research into post-traumatic stress responses in residents losing their homes in Gaza.

This reminds us that some crises involve not just individuals but communities and even whole countries. These crises include those experienced when major catastrophic events occur requiring coordination of services (Raphael, 1986; Hodgkinson and Stewart, 1991; Newburn, 1996). The horrors of individual and community tragedies are repeated on a global scale with famine, floods, fires, epidemics, earthquakes, tsunami, mass murder, transport and technology accidents and terrorism (Hong Chui and Ford, 2000). All are devastating reminders of the unpredictability of natural phenomena or of human frailty. Since 11 September 2001 in the United States, 7 July 2005 in England and the many related incidents worldwide, the awareness of both the potential for disaster and trauma and awareness of the diversity of grief reactions has heightened.

The definitions of disaster imply extraordinary seriousness and great human suffering. However there are many overlapping characteristics relevant to both crisis and catastrophe: both are marked by rapid time sequences, disruption of usual coping responses, perceptions of threat and helplessness, major changes in behaviour and a turning to others for help (Raphael, 1986). Similarly, personal tragedies such as the loss of a loved one by violent means or someone who has been diagnosed with a terminal illness will produce reactions such as shock, disbelief, denial, magical thinking, depersonalisation, sleep disorders, depression, anger, guilt and isolation. Sudden death or losses of any kind produce syndromes characteristic of disaster responses.

The time phases of disaster include:

threat – impact – taking stock of the effects – rescue and recovery

and resemble those of crisis reactions, though there tends to be post-disaster euphoria at having survived and immediate convergence from far and wide to help the stricken community. Nevertheless, the predominant need for people in states of crisis and those affected by disaster is for *information* by which to make meaning of such overpowering experiences, seeking to understand by describing what happened, and trying to restore some sense of command over the powerlessness, which the very thought of extraordinary destruction brings.

Reflections on the various catastrophic events have revealed that there can be long-term psychological effects of trauma, and that early counselling of survivors, bereaved relatives and friends and those in the rescue services can prevent pathological outcomes in the years that follow. As a result, teams of counsellors are made available to those who have had direct experience of a disaster. However, the outpourings of grief from the public at the death of Princess Diana in 1997 and similar public deaths are also indicative of another phenomenon. Even when people have not directly experienced loss at a particular time, public deaths or attending the funeral of others less well known to us can remind us of other more personal losses and precipitate unresolved grief reactions.

When setting up post-disaster aftercare those involved in counselling the survivors need to be both appropriately trained and have an appropriate infrastructure for support.

There are many different ways in which survivors attempt to gain command in the immediate post-disaster phase. These can include:

- *Talking through*, putting into words (and therefore outside oneself), the meaning of the experience. However, someone who tells his or her story again and again with no emotional abreaction can become locked into the experience.
- *Giving testimony*, wanting to write about or talk on the media about the process is a further attempt to gain control over the events and to guide others in the future. Such testimony has also led to people becoming actively involved in campaigning to help prevent the situations that led to the disaster recurring. The involvement of the parents of children killed in shootings in the anti-gun lobby is just one example of this.
- *Feelings* are often the most difficult to release, perhaps only coming later when the catastrophe is safely behind. Long after impact, sensory perceptions may remain as frightening memories. For instance, the awful noise accompanying any event or the terrible silence and stillness, vivid visual experiences and the smell of the disaster haunt those who

survived the terrorist attacks on the Twin Towers in New York in September 2001.

- *Tears* are important in the release of feelings, may be triggered by others' grief and distress, though, as we have said, sometimes difficult for some men or cultures where they are viewed as weakness. Caregivers, such as ambulance personnel, doctors or social workers, are sometimes hidden victims of disasters when they are assumed to be invulnerable. Communal rituals and public acknowledgement of suffering may also help tears and anger, but generally feelings have to come out bit by bit when the person can gradually test out how he/she feels.

- *Perception of the future* and the need to get on with the demands of living is a signal that recovery has started, some trust in the world and hope returns; certain survivors become more aware of what matters to them and have a greater insight into their coping resources (see Raphael, 1986).

As mentioned earlier, care for workers and helpers is an important component of any treatment approach. Psychological debriefing to lessen the stress of encounters with death and devastation prevents illness that can arise out of feelings of depression at not being able to do more. Lack of preparation for the role, whether through lack of training or shock, may mean that those involved require support. Sadly, disasters, attacks and the effects of conflicts and war seem to be more common (or perhaps rolling news makes us more aware of them). There has been an increase in training in counselling skills and counselling is now routinely offered to those immediately affected by the events and who need to unload grief, fear and anger, but this involves intense emotions for workers. Support groups for workers are important, especially when they prevent the helpers feeling that they have failed. Group processes help members to understand their own reactions, reviewing positive and negative aspects in order to integrate (that is, be able to look at a distance and retrospectively) what was learned for oneself, for others and for the future.

Prevention

Preventive work is a neglected aspect of crisis intervention. If there are two types of crisis, those that can be foreseen, such as lifecycle transitions, and those that are accidental or unforeseen, such as sudden bereavement, then there is scope in the former to prepare for the change. Because maturational crises can be anticipated, public health systems that operate services to maintain mental health could be developed to respond to these. Of course, politically, any preventive service is likely to be threatened when there are cutbacks. But it is somewhat short-sighted of social policy planners and social services to simply react to crises on a case-by-case basis.

When tragedies, such as those considered above, occur, many are actually 'human-made', such as wars, traffic accidents and toxic-waste disasters. Here too, preventive action, known as *primary prevention*, is possible, with coordinated services made ready to prevent long-term psychological and other effects. We know that on an individual level, 'anticipatory worry work' helps later grieving, as do ceremonial rituals practised for a long time after a death by some cultures (Raphael, 1984; Parkes, 1986). Services need to be geared to lowering the incidence of mental disorder precipitated by stress or unresolved grief.

Crisis intervention at a *secondary preventive level*, that is, help geared to people who are actually in crisis, is equally at risk from unenlightened policy makers. Preventive work, for example individual counselling, is now being offered predominantly in the independent and private sectors. Anyone can set up as a therapist, charging for services. This means that access to such services is only available to those who have the means to purchase them. It also means that there is no regulation of the provision, or accountability of those offering it.

An important secondary preventive level is in terms of bereavement work relating to terminal illness. Agnew and colleagues (2010) highlight that the challenge for health and social care professionals is to identify individuals who are at risk of lasting physical or mental health problems and to offer bereavement support to reduce the risk of adverse bereavement outcomes. Their research with Marie Curie Cancer Care indicates that while there are ethical issues to consider, the use of bereavement assessments by palliative care social workers can assist in identifying people who need specialist intervention at the point of their bereavement. In this context it is vital that social workers work alongside colleagues in specialist health care to ensure an appropriate response to individual need.

As we have seen, help given at the right time, when a person is psychologically amenable, can prevent long-term development of any of these systems. Fortunately, some recognition of how we can set up *tertiary prevention* services (the help given to those people who have actually been made worse by earlier intervention), can be seen in the efforts to re-establish long-term patients from psychiatric hospitals back in the community. Community development approaches, discussed in Chapter 11, could provide the opportunity to practise primary, preventive crisis intervention, not simply by putting right harmful interventions but by intervening in ways to counteract destructive forces that affect mental health.

Conclusion

This chapter has described how research and practice have helped identify the range of emotions that occur in reaction to crises, either developmental crises or those involving trauma and sudden loss. It identifies that many of these reactions are normal and understandable and that staying with people while they experience them is an important skill. In discussing different models of crisis, reaction and grief it acknowledges that aspects of diversity and different theoretical positions inform understandings of how to work with people in crisis, whatever has precipitated that crisis.

Practice focus

Tom, aged 32, is a soldier who had served in the Iraq war where he had confronted the deaths and disfiguring injuries of others, although he had been physically unharmed. On returning home stressors such as words or places brought back all the intensity of the violence. This was not helped by the fact that discussion of the continuing fighting was frequently in the media. He had recurrent dreams of the events, was hyper alert and gradually became irritable and aggressive with his family.

When he had first returned home, he and his family were elated that he had survived and returned. After several weeks his family expected him to get on with living and to 'put it all behind him'. Unfortunately, Tom could not do this – encountering violent death for the first time in his life he was preoccupied with death and the war. After a time, no one wanted to listen to him and he buried the intrusive images of his experiences.

He even shut out the fact that he had been exposed to the killing of his closest comrade. So effective was his denial that he joined with the other soldiers to rejoice when the attack was over; this psychic numbness helped him through, protecting him from what is dreadful about war – that killing may be necessary for personal survival. It stopped the feeling then, and he continued to block it out on his return home. On discharge he continued to protect his ego, his defence against death anxiety and guilt. Because his family, relieved that he was safe, did not want to listen to his accounts he became isolated, depressed and withdrawn, and was referred to mental health workers skilled in treating post-traumatic stress disorder.

Tom was helped in abreactive sessions, that is, to try to remember the blur of events on the day that his friend was killed. In a group, he and other survivors drew on their anger and their pain in order to externalise their feelings about traumatic events. After some weeks, Tom was helped to face the detail of what had happened on the day of loss, what he had been doing and so on in detail. A breakthrough occurred when he was able to shed tears for the first time. Like other people who want to give testimony to what the experience meant and how others may gain from it, Tom wrote about his recovery. His account begins: I think now that at last the war is over for me, though it will always be there for me for the rest of my days. Looking back I have come to realise that we fight our battles on two fronts; one against the enemy in our sights, the other against the enemy within ourselves'.

Point for reflection

Asking people to undertake exercises related to grief, bereavement and crises is difficult. Working with crises can precipitate feelings associated with our own losses. It is for this reason that it is important for workers to be aware of ways in which they may be affected by their own experiences. This can help bring new insights as well as avoiding blocks. What follows therefore are some ways of reflecting on our own strengths and vulnerabilities.

1 Experiencing loss. Think about a time when you lost something. This can be as simple as losing your keys or your diary or you may choose to focus on a more significant loss. The choice is yours. Write down all the experiences you went through and divide these up into:
   - 'somatic' reactions: that is, physical bodily reactions;
   - 'emotional' or some say 'psychic' reactions: that is, how we feel and what we think;
   - behavioural reactions: what we do.

This analysis might help illustrate some of the theories related to crisis, grief and bereavement discussed in this chapter.

2 *Coping with loss.* If you feel able to focus now on a more significant loss. Again you should choose something that you feel able to think and talk about. Using a tape recorder, tell yourself how you coped with this loss. That is describe to the tape recorder, using sentences starting with, for example, 'I did ...', I felt ...', what you did, how you felt, and so on. This is 'telling yourself' because only you will listen to the tape.

Listen to the tape recorder. What do the words you use tell you about the way you felt about the experience? If you feel able, listen to the tape recorder again and again looking out for different things. For example, what seem to be the significant things that helped you cope? How much did you share with other people?

These exercises will help you to reflect on how you have coped with loss and this will provide strength for you when dealing with other people's loss. However remember that this might be a difficult or painful experience for you. You should ensure that if it becomes too difficult you stop the exercise and talk with someone else – a close friend, a tutor or a counsellor if you feel that would help. Such self-reflection and the ability to recognise painful areas is an indication of strength.

Putting it into practice

This chapter argues that both individual workers and organisations should have the resources to deal with crisis, loss and bereavement either in individual work or in organisational structures. In your practice try and find out if this is so:

1 Ask for details of organisation policies to respond to disasters.
2 Talk with colleagues about their own training and their own work. Do they think they use crisis theory? Are they undertaking bereavement work?
3 In the locality try and identify what other organisations are available to deal with people in crisis, such as Rape Crisis, Cruse. If you were in need of such help how easy would it be to locate these?

Messages from research

Agnew, A. et al. (2010) 'Bereavement Assessment Practice in Hospice Settings: Challenges for Palliative Care Social Workers', *British Journal of Social Work*, describes a qualitative research project into bereavement practice in ten Marie Curie hospices across the UK. The findings have informed the development of a post-bereavement service model that has been subsequently implemented across Marie Curie Cancer Care.

Further resources

Graves, D. (2009) *Talking with Bereaved People: an approach for structured and sensitive communication*, London: Jessica Kingsley. This gives guidance about how to talk with someone who has been bereaved. It deals with some of the theoretical developments in the field of death, dying and bereavement and shows how they can inform everyday practice.

Sapey, B. (2004) 'Impairment, disability, and loss: reassessing the rejection of loss', *Illness, Crisis & Loss*, 12(1), pp. 90–101 provides an excellent overview of theories of loss and bereavement and the implications of these for older people and people with disabilities.

Sheldon, F. (1997) *Psychosocial Palliative Care: good practice in the care of the bereaved and dying*. Cheltenham: Stanley Thornes. This is an excellent introduction to the theory, practice and emotions involved in working with those experiencing loss through terminal illness.

The National Institute for Clinical Excellence (NICE, 2004) guidance on cancer services *Improving Supportive and Palliative Care for Adults with Cancer* recommends a three-component model of bereavement, aimed at ensuring that individual needs are addressed through appropriate levels of service provision (pp. 160–1).

There are UK wide documents providing advice and guidance on end-of-life and bereavement which contain basic principles, standards and elements considered necessary in developing bereavement services:

Department of Health (2005) 'When a patient dies: advice on developing bereavement services in the NHS', London, Department of Health, available online at: http://www.dh.gov.uk/prod_consum_ dh/groups/dh_digitalassets/edh/een/documents/digitalasset/ ,dh_4122193.pdf (accessed 11 May 2010).

Department of Health (2008) 'End of life care strategy: promoting high quality care for all adults at the end of life', London, Department of Health, available online at: ww.dh.gov.uk/en/Publicationsand statistics/Publications/PublicationsPolicyAndGuidance/DH_086277.

Department of Health, Social Services and Public Safety (DHSSPS) (2009) Northern Ireland Health and Social Care Services Strategy for Bereavement Care, Belfast, DHSSPS, available online at: www.dhsspsni.gov.uk/nihsc-strategy-for-bereavementcare-june-2009.pdf.

CHAPTER 8

Problem solving practice

Introduction

It could be argued that all social work is about problem solving. This chapter discusses specific ways of working with individuals to find solutions to their problems that have evolved over time. While the most well established approach has been associated with the well-specified set of procedures of task-centred practice in recent years other approaches have been developed. These concentrate on solving immediate problems rather than trying to identify the cause. Solution-focused practice has therefore been associated with empowering approaches to social work.

All problem solving approaches start from the premise that people come to social work agencies, or are referred to them, because they want their situation improved, they have problems that need solving. To spend time trying to analyse people and social situations is therefore not always appropriate not least because it can sometimes be oppressive by implying that the person is at fault and/or responsible for their problems.

Task-centred practice

Prior to the 1960s, social work practitioners tended to concentrate less on problem solving processes and more on in-depth assessment and the client–worker relationship. Models of practice tended to involve long-term work; exploration of clients' feelings; a tendency to talk about, rather than take action on, difficulties and an interest in underlying, rather than presenting problems. This meant cases were kept open indefinitely: visiting was done on a friendly but aimless basis; providing services was the global aim but there were few specific goals to be accomplished, with or without the clients' agreement. Social work was said to be more about 'maintenance mechanics' than change (Davies, 1985). Proponents of problem solving practice propose that social work should be a focused activity leading to change and, in doing so, should educate clients to become good at problem solving themselves.

The significant contribution made by task-centred practice is that it moves workers from individualised therapeutic approaches to problem solving techniques. It acknowledges that the person with the problem also has the means to resolve it, and that social work intervention should become more of a partnership. It can therefore be seen as a method that empowers users of social work services.

As the various names suggest (e.g. brief intervention, planned short-term treatment) task-centred practice is focused work, which is time limited and offers approaches to problem solving, that takes into account both the needs of individuals to bring about change in their situations, and the requirements of agencies that work should be targeted and effective. It has maintained its popularity through changes in social work (Doel, 2002). It complements other approaches while at the same time being seen as a method of intervention in its own right. It is a method that has been tried and tested in a wide variety of agencies and is both derived from research and lends itself to research (Ford and Postle, 2001). More importantly it has proved effective with a range of problems and with people from diverse cultures and backgrounds.

Students sometimes confuse the task-centred approach with crisis intervention (described in the previous chapter) because both encompass time-limited, focused work and both may be used when service users are temporarily unable to sort out their own problems and are better able to use help to improve coping in a time-limited framework. This is as far as the similarity goes. Turbulent change can occur in crises which call for worker responsiveness that is not necessarily goal directed. People in crisis usually cannot easily conceptualise their problems or the solutions without fairly heavy dependency on the worker in the initial and mid-way stages. In addition, those in crisis are not ready for an energetic, problem solving, equitable relationship with a worker. Nor are they able to agree to a detailed contract that needs to be carefully thought through and planned. Finally the ending in task-centred work is predetermined rather than dependent on the psychological recovery of the person in crisis. In sum, people in crisis are unlikely to be able to cope with the demands of a fully task-centred approach.

Background to the task-centred approach

The initial research study (Reid and Shyne, 1969) that led to the development of task-centred work involved an experimental brief service of Planned Short-Term Treatment (PSTT). It compared this with the usual practice in the agency of long-term service lasting up to eighteen months. To everyone's surprise, the clients in the short-term group improved more than those given the continued service. In fact the latter tended to deteriorate!

The researchers hypothesised that a law of diminishing returns was operating. They suggested that, for both workers and clients, the closer a deadline the more motivated we become. Once help is extended beyond a certain point, clients may lose confidence in their own ability to cope (as intimated in crisis intervention) and become dependent on the worker or the agency and they may develop a kind of unhelpful attachment. In addition, when improvement or change does occur it is likely to occur early on in 'treatment', regardless of the worker's implicit long-term goals.

In recent years another set of theoretical assumptions have come to underpin the use of a task-centred approach. Emancipatory approaches that draw on constructivist understandings have become fundamental to good social work practice. As discussed in Chapter 2 on assessment, constructivism means that social workers have to work with the situation as it is understood by the person experiencing it, rather than imposing their own constructions and interpretations on it. This understanding also has to inform the way that the situation is dealt with. In task-centred practice the service user and worker have to work with the shared understanding of the problem.

The development of a specific task-centred 'therapy' (this now seems a contradiction in terms) based on the results of research (Reid and Epstein, 1972) led to a goal-directed framework. This is why Cree and Myers (2008) argue that task-centred social work is more a model than a theory. The framework involved a maximum of twelve interviews within three months, focusing on limited, achievable goals chosen by the client. The framework was refined by observing its use in practice (Reid and Epstein, 1977). This refinement has continued with Reid developing a guide to task 'menus' (see Doel, 2002, p. 195) and the publication of *The Task-Centred Book* (Marsh and Doel, 2005).

Research in the UK (Goldberg *et al.*, 1977) also helped refine the approach. This found that the model applied to only a minority of clients at least in its 'pure' form. Those with a need for practical resources, who acknowledged that they had a problem, fared best. Involuntary/unwilling clients or those who had chronic, complex problems were less amenable. It was also found that tackling small, manageable objectives, rather than vague global ones, proved more realistic. For example, it is not helpful to set up a contract that requires someone to stop offending. This is both a negative way of putting things (doing something positive is preferred), and it is unrealistic. Working with a young person, who is persistently offending, to identify what s/he needs to do to help them desist from offending would be more positive, and more manageable. This might involve being involved in organised activities or spending leisure time in more purposeful ways.

Further UK research (Goldberg *et al.*, 1985) suggested clients who could not be helped included those whose lifestyle centred round chronic 'cliff-hanging' episodes and those whose difficulties were deep-seated and longer term. Other groups who were identified as not likely to respond to a task-centred approach were those not in touch with reality, for example people involved in substance abuse and those with severe mental disorders.

The task-centred approach

Research indicates that task-centred practice can be used to deal with *eight problem areas* (which cover most of the referrals met with by practitioners). They are:

- interpersonal conflict
- dissatisfaction in social relations
- problems with formal organisations
- difficulties in role performance
- problems of social transition
- reactive emotional distress
- inadequate resources
- behavioural problems. (Reid, 1978; Reid and Hanrahan, 1981)

There are definite steps to be taken in the process of problem solving. These are *five phases* or steps to be taken in helping clients to achieve their own goals:

1. *Problem exploration* or entry – when clients' concerns are elicited, clarified, defined in explicit terms and ranked in order of importance to the client. In certain circumstance (for example where there is a court order) there may be mandated problems and/or tasks.
2. *Agreement* is reached with the client on the target for change, which is then classified by the worker under the previous eight categories. In this stage sometimes problems can be confused with goals. For example not having somewhere to live can be framed as a problem but finding somewhere to live is a goal.
3. *Formulating an objective* that has been decided jointly. Agreement is reached on the frequency and duration of the working (not legal) contract which clarifies respective tasks and roles. The tasks to be undertaken do not always have to involve 'physical doings' but they can include tasks such as cognitive reflections (Doel, 2002).
4. *Achieving the task(s)*, for which no prescribed methods or techniques are proposed within task-centred literature.
5. *Termination* is built in from the beginning. When reviewing the achievements, the worker's efforts are examined, not merely those of the client or the other helping networks.

Some techniques in each of the five phases

Once again, these are not recipes for action, merely some notion of what is likely to crop up in the sequence of phases towards problem resolution.

Phases 1 and 2
In the initial contact, exploration and agreement phases (say between one and six contacts), if the client is not self-referred:

- find out what the referrer's goals are;
- negotiate specific goals and if these can be time-limited;
- negotiate with the referrer what resources they will offer to achieve these goals.

If the client applies independently and voluntarily:

- encourage the client to articulate their problems;
- encourage ventilation of feelings about these;
- step in with immediate practical help if necessary;

- assist the person to take some action on their own, something small and achievable;
- elicit the array of problems with which the client is currently concerned;
- explain how the task-centred approach works, for example, time limits;
- priority focus; schedule for interviews; anyone else who needs to be involved, such as family member;
- define the stated problems in specific, behavioural terms;
- tentatively determine target problems with client;
- choose a maximum of three problems ranked for priority by the client;
- classify the problems under the eight categories; and
- list the problems in a written contract, if used.

Phases 3 and 4
In formulating objectives and achieving the tasks (say between the fourth and tenth contact):

- make the task selection phase short, if the targeting of problems has been done carefully – this will indicate what/who needs to change;
- get the client to think out her/his own tasks and what effects will be likely, helping if the client's assessment looks unrealistic, will make things worse or cannot be achieved in the time;
- if other people are involved, get their agreement too;
- if need be, help the client to generate alternatives and identify what resources are around;
- support task performance by a variety of problem solving means – for instance, refer to a specialised source if this is required (e.g. debt counselling, vocational guidance, classes to learn a language), demonstrate or use games/simulations/video; rehearse problem solving, report back how it went, accompany client for moral support, discuss client's fears, plans, resources, regularly record the status of the problem, examine obstacles and failures in detail;
- if other areas of concern emerge, decide in collaboration with the client if these are worth pursuing;
- always ask about all the tasks in case failures are not mentioned;
- if the method has been modified as partially task-centred (for example for assessment only or time limits are not part of the

contract) consider what follow-up or alternatives will be used.

Phase 5
In the termination (hard to predict how long the process takes in each situation but, say, the final two to three contacts):

- talk about what will be the effect of ending the contact;
- find ways of helping clients to cope with anxieties;
- review progress and give encouragement;
- help clients to identify further areas of work;
- extend time limits only if clients feel that they need extra time and have shown commitment to working on tasks;
- monitor only when mandated by agency or legal requirements or if part of a community care 'package';
- evaluate each person's inputs and record outcomes;
- say goodbye sensitively.

Throughout all of these phases, workers have to draw on skills discussed in the first part of this book. Communication has to be both systematic and responsive and requires both directive and non-directive approaches. Combining these skills with a structured use of time and planned strategies helps to accomplish change in a step-by-step fashion. A fundamental principle is not to judge the person and to ensure that the focus for the task-centred work is *agreed* by both service user and worker, and not imposed by the worker's interpretation of 'what the real problem is'.

Framework for understanding task-centred practice

Effective task-centred practice, however, requires understanding not only what has to be done, but also, why. This is not about trying to analyse the cause of problems in order to work on them, but more about knowing what makes the method effective. Critical reflection on each piece of work will help workers understand more about what has contributed to its success or failure. In this way workers can mirror what they need to do when they are using the method, as the purpose of task-centred work is to provide a form of training session for service users, helping them to discover what works and does not work for them (Doel, 2002).

A synthesis of the characteristics of the method includes:

- *Theories* that underlie the task-centred practice are really only concepts: they include the crisis notion that focused help given at the right time is as effective as long-term service. Also, task accomplishment is viewed as an essential process in human coping endeavours, the choice of tasks and success in tackling them motivates people towards improved problem solving. Becoming effective in certain situations strengthens the ego; success breeds success.

- *Problems* are psychosocial in nature. Having said that, this does not mean that they rest in the individual but that there is a subtle relationship between the individual's experience of the problem and the structural circumstances in which the problem is situated. This relationship is evident in the way that the person constructs or describes the problems.

- *Goals* are modest, achievable, specific and often framed in behavioural terms; they are chosen by the client in collaboration with the worker. Goals are inherent in each of the five phases, completion of which would qualify the approach as fully task-centred. However, a partially task-centred approach is possible when only some of these phases are reached: an example of this would be task-centred assessment.

- *The client's role* is to identify desirable and feasible goals and to specify tasks and sub-tasks, prioritised in a working agreement with the social worker.

- *The worker's role* is to make explicit the time limits to the client and the agencies involved and to assist in the problem search, target and task-setting by which problems are reduced and some solutions found.

- *Techniques* include: problem specification; task planning; analysing obstacles; structuring interview time; reviewing and ending.

Practice focus

Mr Singh was a sixty-seven-year-old widower. He had spent his adult life in England but his work had involved travelling which meant he has no friends in the locality in which he eventually settled. His married sons, who lived many miles away, only visit him two or three times a year. Following a stroke, Mr Singh has been accommodated in a facility for disabled people, but during the six months he has been there he has become reclusive and uncooperative. Rehabilitation efforts had ceased because staff complained that Mr Singh was unmotivated and aggressive; they even wondered if he was clinically depressed, as he slumped all day in a wheelchair, keeping himself to himself.

The social worker received a referral from the care staff to sort out the numerous debts that had accrued because Mr Singh had not claimed any benefits. She found that, far from being hostile, Mr Singh was a gentle, shy man who was not used to discussing his private affairs. She also considered that there were cultural differences in the way that Mr Singh might react to strangers knowing about his personal affairs. Culture might also affect the way that Mr Singh reacted to female carers.

The social worker suggested that they try to deal with his debts by using a task-centred approach. This would focus on what needed to be done, not pry into Mr Singh's background. He seemed more able to talk about concrete problems which he described as 'problems with formal organisations' and 'inadequate resources'. His goal was to become more independent. The contract was agreed that they would meet weekly to work on two target problems:

1 To pay off rent, telephone and fuel bills within the following three months.
2 To claim outstanding benefits from social security, insurance companies and salary from previous employers.

General tasks, such as writing letters, listing the debts, making phone calls and deciding who would do what were dealt with in the first two meetings. A schedule was drawn up about the frequency and duration of the meetings (mornings and for twenty-five minutes as Mr Singh tired easily). They agreed also to let the centre staff know what would happen.

Every Monday the social worker discussed with Mr Singh how the debts could be cleared and which were the most pressing. Responsibilities were allocated and each week they reviewed each other's task accomplishments. Sometimes the worker had to obtain necessary forms and give Mr Singh assistance in completing them. This was, in part, because, although Mr Singh was fluent in spoken English, the technical language of the forms was not always easy to understand. Although there were minor changes to what was initially agreed no revision of the contract was needed.

Mr Singh, in one of the task-centred discussions, confided to the worker his fear of returning home to live alone, and his loneliness at not knowing any neighbours. He talked about his shyness that had even stopped him getting to know anyone in the unit. He also recognised that he would like to be able to share with people from his own cultural background. Accepting that he had overcome his shyness with the worker, they examined ways in which to start a conversation, re-negotiating a further task-centred working agreement that:

1 He would start a conversation with one of his companions at lunch every day.
2 He would write to his sons telling them how he had sorted out his finances, and ask if they would visit him some time.

Because Mr Singh became more outgoing, physiotherapy and occupational therapy were restarted, resulting in him being able to try walking with a tripod. One of Mr Singh's sons made a visit and offered to have his father home with him for a period to assess if this could be a long-term arrangement.

The benefits of undertaking task-centred practice

First, and most importantly, although task-centred practice offers a specific set of procedures, where service users are helped to carry out problem-alleviating tasks within agreed periods of time, it does not mean simply assigning tasks, or setting 'homework', such as is common in behavioural and family therapies. Tasks are not just activities; they have meaning because of the overall structure in which they take place. The person is the main change agent, helping the worker to assess and choose what the priorities for change ought to be and then agreeing who is going to do what. The movement from problem to goal is by tasks which are as diverse and varied as the problems, goals, users and services that generate them (Marsh, 2002).

Task-centred practice is useful at initial referral stage in a single agency but interdisciplinary teams set up to establish community care may also use a form of task-centred practice, basing their shared goals on what is worked out with service users, in addition to having a pre-planned exit time.

Debate has taken place about the use of task-centred work in work that has been mandated by the courts, specifically in criminal justice work. Aspects of the method have been adopted by Trotter (2006) in his work with 'involuntary clients' discussed in the next chapter. However, the nature of the problems presented by offenders, in that they may be out of touch with reality by virtue of substance abuse or mental disorder, sometimes mean that this method is not appropriate.

Any practice which ensures that there is no misunderstanding about why contact is taking place is likely to be more successful – if only because it is more honest and does not build up false expectations. It also means that where the social worker is acting as an agent of social control, or is intent upon offering protection; there is no ambiguity about this.

Many social work methods have been experienced as eurocentric (Milner and O'Byrne, 2002). However, as can be seen from the case study, task-centred practice requires that the worker actively embraces diversity and considers the implications of culture on the problems experienced, how they are communicated and the methods used to solve them. The methods do not further oppress people by taking over their lives or implying that the worker knows best. There is no mystery about what the worker is doing because s/he is as accountable as the service users in carrying out agreed tasks. This lessens the sense of powerlessness when faced with 'authority' figures.

Apart from the somewhat rigid time limits, which possibly ignore certain ethnic traditions which prefer more gradual introduction of 'strangers' into family and community relations, task-centred work is beneficial in working with different cultures in that it:

1. Takes into account not only individual but also collective experiences during the stages of problem search, agreement and setting tasks. The source of the problem is not presumed to reside in the client; as much attention is paid to external factors, such as welfare rights and housing, where there is scope for supplying 'power' resources such as information and knowledge. The role for the worker is one of resource consultant.
2. Focuses on individuals, couples, families, groups and/or organisations. Practical advice on how to approach problems and systems can be rehearsed, modified and copied in groups; peers, as well as social workers, can act as teacher/trainers in problem solving (Marsh and Doel, 2005).
3. Addresses the strengths of people and their networks. For instance, it is an antidote to the process of labelling, which assumes that being black, Asian or other ethnic group is a problem. There is scope to valorise strengths of different ethnic groups and use the resources of their particular communities (Ahmad, 1990). One aim of the method is to enhance self-esteem as well as problem solving.

4. Provides positive feedback for people who are not used to success. Setting achievable goals and do-able tasks means that people are more likely to fulfil them. The goals also have to be something to which the service user is motivated. Even though achieving the ultimate goal might take time, identifiable progress towards a desired goal provides motivation for further success.
5. Does not rely on the notion of self-disclosure via a one-way, vertical helping relationship, it tries to put worker and client on the same footing.

Solution-focused practice

In many ways, solution-focused approaches in social work seem similar to task-centred work in that they both concentrate on the problem not the person, try to resolve difficult and complex situations, and both are forward looking. Many of the benefits identified above are also relevant in solution-focused approaches. However there are differences, both in the underpinning rationale and in the practicalities of the method.

O'Connell (2004, p. 21) provides a useful analysis of the differences between task-focused and solution-focused approaches. The limitations of task-centred practice are that people have to be quite robust to respond to the method. Solution-focused is located directly in a strengths-perspectives approach arguing that, even in the most complex and desperate situations, personal resources of the service user can be found and built on. Another difference is that task-centred work involves the worker *helping* the service user identify realistic goals while solution-focused work depends on the service user's hopes and dreams, even if these are unrealistic (Cree and Myers, 2008). Solution-focused work grew out of research on labelling and stigma (Healy, 2005) and also relates to work on resilience (see Chapter 9). However, the underpinning approach or theory is that of a strengths perspective.

Strengths-based approaches

Initially based on a project for users of mental health services (Saleeby, 1996), a strengths-based approach identifies that:

• The focus of the helping process is upon consumers' strengths, interests and abilities; not upon their weaknesses, deficit or pathologies.

- People with mental illness can learn, grow and change.
- The consumer is viewed as the director of the helping process.
- The consumer–care manager relationship becomes the indispensable foundation for mutual collaboration.
- Assertive outreach is the preferred mode of working with consumers.

While the terminology is different (note the use of consumer, not client or service user) this approach is seen to resonate with social work, drawing on the values of both individualisation and empowerment. It starts from the premise that there is always something working in peoples lives and that service users have under-utilised resources to deal with problems, therefore they have potential (Hogg and Wheeler, 2004). It, therefore, is an optimistic approach, which focuses on the service users' capabilities and potential (Healy, 2005) and as such, is associated with empowerment. The approach has now been extended to other service user groups.

Aspects of a solution-focused approach, based on a strengths perspective, are that the problem is depersonalised and that working together the worker and the service user are involved in a mutual learning process, the worker does not have all the answers. Finally an overarching principle is that the work is forward looking, trying to find future possibilities. As Milner summarises it: 'solution focused therapy constructs solutions rather than deconstructs problems' (Milner, 2000, p. 336).

There are therefore five key assumptions in solution-focused practice. Workers must:

- adopt optimistic attitudes
- focus primarily on assets
- collaborate with the service user
- work towards long-term empowerment
- create community

While these seem grand principles it is important to remember that working with them can create small changes in a service user's situation. This can help the worker to approach situations in a different way and move from a 'vicious circle of problem maintenance' (which some have associated with long-term casework) to a virtuous circle of problem resolution (Hogg and Wheeler, 2004). Situations in which social workers intervene are sometimes described as 'chronic' and service users either remain as an open file on a social worker's workload or they have to keep returning to the social work agency when new 'problems' arise. This very terminology is negative and suggests that people become an administrative and workload burden, rather than individuals or families experiencing challenges with which they need help to resolve, both in the immediate and long-term future. O'Connell describes how workers have to 'change the discourse' (2004, p. 36) to focus on change, solutions and strategies. This does not mean that social workers have to find 'the magic bullet' – the solution to all the problems – all in one go. Working together, the worker and the service user(s) are future oriented. This involves identifying the resources and capabilities of the service user that can help them cope with the current situation, but might also work in future problem situations. The emphasis, therefore, is on what is working in any situation and building strengths rather than repairing deficits (Milner, 2000). However, while having this forward-looking, positive approach it is also important for worker and service user to acknowledge what is not working.

Practice

As in task-centred work, research and practice have identified a number of stages to the practice of solution-focused work. For example Hogg and Wheeler (2004) identify:

- *Goal clarification:* where service users are encouraged to identify outcomes rather than rigidly outline the problems. For example, if a family is living in overcrowded, neglected private accommodation and has not acquired enough points to qualify for local authority provided housing, it does not help them if the worker asks them to merely reiterate what is wrong with the accommodation.
- *Pre-session change:* If the worker conducts an optimistic and forward-looking first interview, it can encourage those identifying the problem to also talk about progress that has been made or positive changes that have occurred. Focusing on this can help identify the resources and approaches that are already being used.
- *Scaling questions:* These are identified as a core tool in solution-focused approaches. Scales are used to help service users identify the extent of the problem: 'On a scale of 1 to 10, how difficult is it to live in your present accommodation?' The scales do not have to be a precise measurement, but help the

service user to explain how difficult the situation is for them, irrespective of what anyone else thinks. Scaling questions can also be used to help identify progress and/or improvement – even small ones. If 10 is the greatest amount of difficulty then 9 is a little less difficult – the positive approach is to identify what has contributed to the reduction. Again, the emphasis is on how the service user perceives the changes.

- *Miracle questions:* This is another core technique to help identify exactly what the service user wants to happen. The miracle question is used to create goals that can be worked towards (Cree and Myers, 2008). It can be framed in a number of ways: 'If a miracle were to happen what changes would you want in your housing situation?'; 'If I had a magic wand and could make the situation better – what would be different?' Hogg and Wheeler (2004) give excellent examples of how this question can be framed in different ways.

- *Exceptions:* A positive forward-looking approach can help identify times when a recurring problem does not happen, or a situation is not so difficult to cope with. This can again help focus on the service user's own resources and coping mechanisms.

- *Compliments*: Core to the positive, strengths-based approach the worker must acknowledge and identify when and how there have been positive changes – or even a positive will to be open about situations and discuss them.

- *Tasks:* From the shared analysis, it is sometimes possible to identify tasks that might be helpful. However, this is done in an empowering way and not part of a 'contract' on which the relationship and future contact is based – which is the nature of tasks in task-centred work.

- *Problem free talk:* When it is appropriate, it is helpful to encourage the service user to talk about times when they were not experiencing this problem. This is not to analyse or deconstruct the problem, but to give them encouragement and raise morale. It also helps sometimes to identify what resources they have drawn on in the past – such as families, friends, etc. Of course this has to be done with care because if it is not right for the service user it might seem to be irrelevant and wasting their time.

These different aspects of solution-focused practice highlight that the method is based on collaboration and capacity building.

The interventions are based on how the service user defines the problem, what they see as the important things to change and identifying what resources they have to bring about that change. These resources might include others: friends, relatives or other professionals. It is this aspect of the work that Healy (2005) identifies as 'creating community'.

To maintain positive focus, workers must draw on their skills of listening, focusing and communicating. This is not too different from other social work approaches but a significant difference, according to Cree and Myers (2008), is that there is no fixed assessment. As more is learnt by the communication and the imagining that grows out of the 'miracle question' the perception of the problem and the recognition of the service user's capabilities changes. Another important feature of this practice is that it concentrates on difference. It acknowledges the uniqueness of the person, how they see the problems they are experiencing and what resources they have to deal with it.

In their research on using this method in an area team, Hogg and Wheeler (2004) found that workers liked the universality of the method. That is because it focuses on differences they found that they could adapt to work with a wide variety of service users – people from all ages, different ethnic and cultural backgrounds and many other aspects of diversity. In fact, the method positively recognises difference. They also found that they could use aspects of the approach in one-off interviews – it did not depend on a whole 'programme' of contacts in the way that task-centred work does.

The limitations of using problem solving practice

So far in this chapter the discussion has been wholly positive and that might suggest that other approaches described in this book are redundant! In fact, Healy (2005) argues that a major strength of solution-focused practice is that it acts as a corrective to other approaches because it challenges what she calls the 'dominant discourse' of worker expertise. It concentrates on the 'social' and not the 'person' and therefore avoids labelling, blaming and stigmatising those who come to social workers for assistance.

However there are limitations to using these methods. The first is relevant to both approaches that have been discussed in this chapter and that is that, even though the focus moves away from the person to the problem, there is still an emphasis on individual solution. This takes no account of the structural causes of problems. For example, the number of people in overcrowded sub-standard housing is because of deficits in local authority house building programmes and a failure to hold private landlords/ladies accountable for the properties they rent out. In some situations, such as housing policy, level of benefit payments, and so on, the solutions do not necessarily rest with the individual who is experiencing the problem but require political action, such as changing local and national policies. Of course, while that political action is being taken the individual and/or the family still have to deal with the impact.

There is a suggestion that in statutory work it is not always possible to work in partnership or to be collaborative because of the power imbalances in the relationship between service user and worker. Interestingly, Cree and Myers (2008) discuss the use of solution-focused practice with offenders. Task-centred practice can be used with offenders on community supervision orders. In criminal justice social work, workers have a great deal of overt power, for example, to take the offender back to court. It is suggested that if the worker can be up-front about the powers that they have and use problem solving methods effectively, then this can help manage the risk of re-offending. Of course, this raises the question of to what extent should social workers focus on the causes of crime, which are outside of the individual?

Criticisms of task-centred practice include concerns that it might lead to workers attempting to pigeon-hole service users, or require them to adopt certain patterns or standards of behaviour. At its worst, task-centred work might be seen as a form of behaviour modification in that only certain forms of problem solving behaviour will be acceptable. Ironically the concerns about solution-focused approaches are that they might be unrealistic or idealistic, raising service users hopes. While these are obvious pitfalls, they can only be avoided by practitioners having appropriate training which leads to an understanding of both the positives and negatives of using the approaches

Both approaches have the advantage of being structured and, in the case of task-centred practice, time limited. The focus on resolution, on outcomes, means that such approaches might be incorporated into managerialist agendas that require rapid throughput of work. Interventions, which are less time consuming for workers, are less costly and it may be this rather than benefits to service users that make them more attractive to organisations. Workers might be encouraged to use such methods because of the need to meet 'targets', such as dealing with cases quickly and reducing waiting lists rather than needs of the service users. Also workers might be pressured to use them as a short-cut or 'quick-fix' solution and ignore the complexities of the situation with which they are faced. Having said that, service users do benefit from focused approaches which address their needs, but this only happens if workers are properly trained in the methods (Hogg and Wheeler, 2004; Marsh and Doel, 2005) and can apply them systematically and without pressure for 'results'.

Conclusion

In looking at methods which concentrate on the problems experienced rather than the person experiencing them this chapter has introduced methods which are seen to be more empowering for service users. Drawing on constructivist approaches detailed in Chapter 2, both task-centred work and solution-focused work try to respond to the needs of services users by drawing on their resources to find solutions to their problems. This does not mean that practical help is not offered and that structural factors that impinge upon individuals and families are not important. However both approaches recognise that social work is not about 'helping' in the sense of doing something *for* or *to* the person; it is about working in partnership with service users, and enabling them to do things for themselves.

Practice focus

Mrs Turner is in touch with Children's Services because her 12-year-old son, Joe, has been demonstrating behavioural difficulties over time. Joe has severe learning disabilities and his frustrations in communicating sometimes cause him to be aggressive. These violent episodes have became more frequent and as Joe is becoming physically bigger and stronger Mrs Turner is less able to calm him in the ways that she had done when he was younger. (She would hold him until his anger subsided.)

Mrs Turner is divorced from her husband. Joe's behaviour had put great strain on the marriage. However Mr Turner is very fond of his son and is in touch with him regularly. Joe attends a local school for children with learning disabilities. He has been 'statemented' but the school wants to call another assessment meeting because Joe's behaviour is deteriorating and they are not sure they can contain him in the school. They say his behaviour is causing difficulties for other children at the school. Mrs Turner agrees Joe's behaviour is getting worse but is concerned that a residential school will be suggested but does not think that this will be good for Joe. She is very tired from looking after Joe alone because Joe's behaviour requires her to do many tasks to 'contain' his behaviour. Mrs Turner feels that if she had more energy she would be more tolerant and able to give Joe more attention and this might help to calm him.

In discussing all aspects of the situation, the social worker asks Mrs Turner the 'miracle' question: what she wants to happen. Ideally Mrs Turner wants Joe not to have learning disabilities, but she knows that this miracle is not going to happen. She loves him dearly and she wants him to continue living with her – she just wants to have more energy to be able to cope. They discuss all the possible ways that this be might achieved and Mrs Turner is asked to 'scale' them. Of all the possibilities she suggests, there is one: as he is so fond of Joe, her ex-husband might be prepared to offer some help. It is agreed that she will raise this with him, and if he is prepared to think about it she will suggest they both meet with the worker.

The joint meeting negotiated arrangements for Joe that involve his father in some of the practical arrangements. Mrs Turner recognises that this might not necessarily be the end of Joe's behavioural problems, but she feels that this will help her to be more able to cope and make decisions on a more rational basis.

Point for reflection

In thinking about the methods discussed in this chapter it is useful to think about what are the positives and negatives of the methods – and what other approaches might have been used.

Both practice examples have very positive endings – but this is not always the case. Thinking about the two examples: consider what could be done if the 'solutions' adopted do not work out. What else could be done using problem solving approaches? What other approaches could be applied in these situations?

Putting it into practice

Choose a situation from practice that seems to have some clear indications that something has to change. Think about how you might use the methods described but remember:

1 The crucial period for problem solving approaches is the early stages of contact. It is important to listen carefully to what is being said about the situation and to discern what the service user says he or she wants changing.

2 You might identify what the service user wants changing by asking the 'miracle' question. It is then important to clarify what has to be done to bring about the necessary change. Remember, tasks need to be small manageable pieces of work that will be undertaken either by the service user or by you.

3 As you identify what needs to change, and work out what has to be done, and who does what it is helpful to write these down – both for yourself and for the service user.

4 Obviously, you will now work with the service user to ensure that you both complete the agreement. However at this point it is also useful to do some reflective work on your own with the agreement. Think about when you first encountered the situation: Does the agreement or contract reflect what you thought about the situation? Would you have chosen to focus on the tasks that the service user has chosen? What do you think the hurdles will be? What do you think are the strengths of the situation?

5 Once you have completed the piece of work with the service user, it is useful to go back to your list and see how the work that developed compared with your assessment. In doing so, try and be honest about how much you influenced the situation and to what extent you were able to let the service user make her/his own decisions.

Messages from research

Task-centred case work was one of the first social work interventions to be researched. The classic study was undertaken by Reid, W. and Shyne, A. (1969) *Brief and Extended Casework*, New York: Columbia University Press in North America. It is interesting to see the use of 'control groups' in this early research.

To test the use of the method (Gibbons *et al.*, 1979) undertook a study also involving control groups. Four hundred people arriving at a hospital casualty department in the UK after taking an overdose were randomly assigned to an experimental task-centred casework service or to the routine aftercare service. In the cases where a task-centred method was used, it proved that people were more satisfied with the service they had received and showed more immediate improvement in social problems than those who had received the routine aftercare service.

Solution focused practice: Corcoran and Pillai (2009) have undertaken a review of research on solution-focused therapy. They searched literature on studies that had been undertaken using 'experimental and quasi-experimental' design, that is, there was some comparison between situations in which the approach was used and those where there was no intervention – although not all the studies involved social work. Of the ten studies that met their criteria, five were deemed to demonstrate that solution-based therapy had some effect but, as this was compared with no intervention, the authors conclude that the effects of solution-focused therapy are equivocal – and that more research is needed in what they describe as a surprisingly under-researched area.

Further resources

Task-centred casework

Doel, M. (2002) 'Task-centred Practice', in Adams, R., Dominelli, L. and Payne, M. (eds) *Social Work: themes issues and critical debates*. Basingstoke: Palgrave Macmilan.
An excellent summary of task-centred work incorporating some new research and development undertaken by one of the originators, William Reid.

Marsh, P. and Doel, M. (2005) *The Task-centred Book*. London: Routledge.

Solution-focused therapy

Myers, S. (2007) *Solution Focused Approaches*. Lyme Regis: Russell House Press.

O'Connell, B. (2004) *Solution Focused Therapy*. London: Sage.
These two texts provide excellent detailed analysis of the theory behind this approach and the detail of how to use it in practice.

Hogg, V. and Wheeler, J. (2004) 'Miracles R them: solution-focused practice in a social services duty team', *Practice*, 16 (4).
A useful article describing the method based on a summary of earlier research and reporting an evaluation of the use of the method by a social work team.

For a useful article written by an ex-social worker now working in a clinical setting and which combines time limited and solution-focused approaches see Iveson, C. (2002) 'Solution-focused brief therapy', *Advances in Psychiatric Treatment*, 8(2), pp. 149–57.

CHAPTER 9

Cognitive-behavioural work

Introduction

The final chapter in this section looks at problem solving methods that have been developed from psychology but which are playing an increasingly important part in social work practice. The basic tenet of behavioural approaches is that behaviour is learned and unlearned. Much of the work was developed in psychology but behaviourism has influenced social work practice in a number of ways. In working with people with learning difficulties, the principles of 'normalisation' or age-appropriate behaviour involve the basic principles of learning theory. Programmes working with offenders, especially those who are dependent upon substances such as drugs or alcohol, have involved cognitive behaviour therapy, as do those working with people experiencing depression.

Background

Behavioural approaches to therapy grew rapidly in the 1950s and 1960s partly to get away from the dominance of the psychoanalytic perspective. One of the significant differences between earlier practice and behavioural work is that those who take a psychosocial approach would say that behaviour, thoughts and attitudes, and feelings are influenced largely by the past and by internal conflict.

In contrast, Skinner (1938), the theorist responsible for developing behaviourism, argued that behaviour and personality are determined mainly by current events in the external environment.

Fundamental to the behaviourist school is the acceptance that if behaviour is learned then it can be unlearned, and new behaviours can be learned. The aim of behaviourist social work is to reduce undesired behaviours and increase desired behaviours. To achieve this cognitive-behavioural therapies (CBT) draw on both learning theory (Sheldon, 2000) and social learning theory (Payne, 2005). There are however different types of learning.

Four types of learning

Psychologists have identified four types of learning, which are basic to an understanding of behavioural therapeutic approaches. *Respondent* (classical) and *operant* conditioning were developed in work with animals. The former explained simple reflex behaviours such as blinking when a light flashes, while the latter model, developed by Skinner (1938), examined non-reflexive, active, trial-and-error learning. Experiments on *observational learning* showed that we also learn by watching other people, while more recent approaches recognise that private self-talk and thoughts govern our behaviour too and contribute to *cognitive learning*.

Respondent conditioning

An example of respondent conditioning was when Pavlov's dogs were taught to salivate at the sound of a tuning fork just before food was presented. The dogs began to respond to the sound of the fork even when there was no food. The stimulus (fork sound) that evoked the response became the conditioned stimulus (S) and the saliva the conditioned response (R). Textbooks represent this as S-R. However, a stimulus might also produce a more generalised response. Hence the *stimulus* (S) of a dog biting an unwary social worker might evoke a fear *response* (R) resulting, perhaps, in the worker avoiding all the places where dogs may lurk (in this event, the dog stimulus has widened and become *generalised* to a fear of all dogs) (Howe, 1987).

In therapy, systematic desensitisation (also called reciprocal inhibition) based on the principle of respondent conditioning, can break the pattern. It is used primarily for anxiety and avoidance reactions. Once the stimuli that provoke anxiety have been assessed, relaxation techniques are taught and the client helped to establish an 'anxiety hierarchy'. So, for example, a person who is afraid to leave the house will be asked to rank which situations he/she finds easy and which most difficult when trying to go outdoors. While the client relaxes, each situation, say from putting out the milk bottles to going to the shops, is imagined progressively up the 'ladder' of feeling. Social workers working with school phobia might use this approach. They may help a pupil to return to school by gradually getting him or her used to the bus route, the playground and finally the classroom with the other children.

Operant conditioning

This consists of actions that operate on the environment to produce consequences. The key feature is that behaviour is altered by its consequences. If the changes brought about by the behaviour are reinforcing (that is, bring about a reward or eliminate something unpleasant for the person) then there is more chance that that behaviour will occur again. Early laboratory experiments involved teaching rats to press a lever to obtain food.

Operant behaviour therapy has been useful in working with people with learning disabilities or those not used to living in the community. A token economy system and verbal praise are used to reward desired behaviour such as self-help and social skills and reduce unwanted, bizarre actions. Unlike insight giving and the psychoanalytic approach, this method has also been found appropriate for people who are diagnosed psychotic, since no interpretation of 'why' the behaviour occurs is necessary. (See Sheldon, 1984, for further examples of this method with those who have mental health problems.)

Positive reinforcement, known as the ABC of behaviour (Hudson and Macdonald, 1986), is most useful for social workers. It has been used in work with parents whose children misbehave. Parents find it fascinating to discover that they may inadvertently have been reinforcing the 'wrong' behaviour. Thus, the child screams and gets a sweet to keep him/her quiet: this behaviour is more likely to occur again because of the reward. To understand the sequence of events it is necessary to examine the Antecedents of the Behaviour and its Consequences (ABC). This is shown diagrammatically opposite:

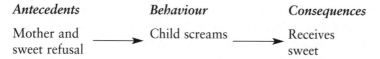

Antecedents	Behaviour	Consequences
Mother and sweet refusal	→ Child screams →	Receives sweet

An important aspect of giving reinforcers, for example in encouraging children in residential accommodation to clear away their games, is that the reward, say a smile or thanks from the staff, should be given *immediately and consistently* by the whole team. This consistent response has to continue until such behaviour is occurring naturally and need not be so systematically commented upon (because the reward tends to lose some of its value over time). Here, 'correct' behaviour is rewarded and undesirable behaviour ignored. Sometimes using a visual aid to record positive gains such as 'star charts' can reward achievements.

Chaining and backward chaining are examples of operant procedures. They can be used to teach new behaviours and have been successful in work with people with learning difficulties (Tsoi and Yule, 1982) or for people who have experienced brain trauma through accident or illness. Teaching self-help skills, such as dressing or brushing one's teeth, is not as simple as it sounds because each successive step to achieve such behaviour has to be separately analysed and progressively tracked. An example of backward chaining was that used by foster parents to teach their foster son, who had a learning difficulty, to make his own bed. The foster mother performed all but the last link in the chain, and then reinforced the child for carrying out the last step of tucking in the sheet. Then the last two links were left for him to accomplish, and so on, backwards. He needed a lengthy programme but eventually gained the satisfaction of fully completing the tasks himself.

The termination of undesired behaviour is called negative reinforcement and is aimed at reinforcing wanted behaviour by deterring unwanted behaviour. Children may learn to keep quiet if only to avoid the pain of being shouted at. This is not to be confused with punishment to deter behaviour, a confusion that has blighted recent social work practice where 'pin down' and other unacceptable procedures have been adopted in residential homes as a means of changing behaviour.

Negative reinforcement is not as welcome as a positive reward because it does little to increase new behaviour, and shouting can sometimes become rewarding when some attention is preferred to none. A combined strategy is more effective if the aim is to decrease or extinguish unacceptable behaviour. Accordingly, when staff in a unit for disabled children wanted to stop a 10-year-old girl from whining, they collectively ignored her when she whined, and played bubbles and gave her a much-loved mirror when she was quiet.

'Time out' (that is, from reinforcement), is an extinction procedure which, when used properly and ethically, can be successful. Some agencies mistakenly control aggressive behaviour by isolating people for lengthy periods – this is not time out but dubious punishment. The procedure should follow within seconds of the misbehaviour, clear explanations should have been given in advance about what would happen and why, and the person should be taken to a time-out area, such as the corner of the room where there are no pleasant distractions or harmful objects for between three and five minutes maximum.

Observational learning

By copying what other people do we can learn something without having to go through a process of trial and error. Bandura (1977) says that there are three different effects of what is known as modelling: we can learn new skills or ideas; social skills can be imitated and practised; and fear responses can be inhibited, for example sitting next to someone on a plane who enjoys the experience. The main difference from the previous two types of learning is that reinforcement is not viewed as essential. Learning can be deliberate, such as the groups set up to teach social skills or assertiveness via role play and video films; or it can be unplanned, when, for instance, service users copy the way workers talk to benefit agency officials on the telephone. Imitative learning is even more likely when there is a good working relationship or where the model is perceived as competent and of high status. This active modelling (pro-social modelling) has been developed by Trotter (2006) as one aspect of work with involuntary clients, and has been used with those in the criminal justice system on court orders. This is discussed in more detail below.

Cognitive learning

Traditionally, learning theory has been concerned with outward behaviour, fixing people as passive beings whose behaviour can be altered by environmental controls. However, it has been recognised by cognitive behaviourists that we also feel and think: we attach meaning to events. For this reason Trevithick (2005a) makes a distinction between cognitive approaches and behaviourist approaches in social work. Beck (1989), working with depressed and emotionally disordered people, suggested that negative thoughts about themselves, their situation and their prospects brought about their emotional disorders.

The idea that thought processes can have an impact on emotions and behaviour is now quite well established. For example Kelly's Personal Construct Theory (Kelly, 1955) showed how people construct their own view of the world, and work is only effective if we can try to understand that view. Ellis's (1962) Rational Emotive Therapy (RET) maintains we are upset not by events but by the view we take of them: we upset ourselves by our irrational thoughts. Modern cognitive-behaviour therapy incorporates ideas from Kelly and Ellis.

Some techniques and procedures

The different approaches to learning mean that there are various ways of changing behaviour; and an increasing number of response options (that is, new skills) are employed by those using a behavioural approach. It is an action-oriented approach. People are helped to take a specific action to change observable behaviour; goals are spelled out in concrete terms and the procedure is almost scientifically evaluated by questioning what was done, how often, by whom, for what specific problem and under which particular circumstances. In the cognitive field, private or subjective meanings are the key to a person learning to understand how his or her cognitions (thoughts) have distorted reality and how, therefore, the individual has the responsibility and the capacity to unravel disturbances, regardless of their origin.

Despite the fact that behaviourist approaches were introduced as a reaction to a psychosocial approach there are various comparisons to be made. Trevithick's (2005a, pp. 260–5) helpful discussion of these comparisons includes: the client selects goals; the relationship is seen as important but not sufficient to achieve change; work is a joint effort; a written plan of action may be signed and the worker functions typically as a teacher who helps the client to understand the method to perpetuate self-help.

The initial stage of work is a behavioural assessment. The implications for assessment are vital because without a baseline the effectiveness of the intervention cannot be judged (Milner and

O'Byrne, 2002). Hence, assessment involves a detailed account of exactly what happens before, during and after a problematic event. The client may keep a diary so that all the factors that could affect outcomes are taken into account. Next, the client says which behaviour is to be increased/decreased. The worker clarifies who or what else in the environment could assist or prevent the change effort (for instance sometimes a partner might subtly reinforce a woman's drinking pattern; slippery floors and high toilets can deter frail elderly people from using the toilet). Each goal is framed in behavioural terms: as with task-centred practice, it is insufficient to say something like, 'John will do as his parents tell him'. Far better to state that John will be home by 9 pm during the week and 10 pm at weekends, what the reward will be and what will happen if he arrives later.

A handout or explanatory leaflet may sustain the person's efforts. For example, in challenging depressive thoughts a client may complete a sheet recording thoughts; the emotions these aroused; the automatic dysfunctional thought that accompanied this, such as 'I am worthless'; what rational thought response he or she tried and the degree of success he or she achieved. Or it could be that the strategy is to increase a person's behavioural repertoire; for instance helping to assert oneself with an authority figure. The techniques would follow the following steps:

1. Identify what behaviour is to be learned.
2. Instruct or demonstrate what this behaviour looks like.
3. Ask the person to role-play or copy the behaviour.
4. Provide feedback and reward desired responses.
5. Rehearse and practise again, modelling again if necessary.
6. Desired behaviour may need to be shaped gradually using praise.
7. Assign homework – 'practice makes perfect'.
8. Evaluate 'before and after' ratings of the behaviour.

This focused and programmatic approach could be seen to challenge the mystique of a psychosocial approach, but overall it does little to move us away from a 'treatment' model.

The growth of cognitive-behaviour therapy

As stated earlier, the field of cognitive-behaviour therapy owes much to the work of Kelly (1955). The basic premise is that we each bring 'theories' about the world, unique ways of anticipating events and relationships, which colour our cognitive processes. Ellis's (1962) work attempted to show that people's aberrations in thinking, such as self-defeating beliefs, create disturbances in the way we feel about things. Ellis would propose that if someone is unhappy after a divorce, it is not the divorce itself that causes this but the person's beliefs about being a failure or losing a partner, or whatever. Beck's application of these ideas to treating depression (see Beck, 1989) in the 1970s contributed significantly to the growth of the cognitive-therapy movement.

By developing a system of psychotherapy that helped people to overcome their blocks and the way they reacted to situations, Beck educated them to understand their cognitive styles and underlying cognitive structures (or unconscious philosophies) that were activated by particular events. Methods to correct erroneous beliefs included:

- An *intellectual* approach, which identified misconceptions, tested how valid these were and then substituted more appropriate concepts.
- An *experiential* approach, which motivated people to experience situations powerfully, which could modify assumptions, and a behavioural approach which encouraged the development of new coping techniques, for instance, systematic desensitisation procedures described earlier.

So Beck worked not only on clients' thoughts, but also on outward behaviour and feelings. More recently the approach has been developed effectively in work with perpetrators of domestic violence, where male 'theories' of women and women's behaviour have been challenged (Macrae and Andrews, 2000).

Most practitioners use the term cognitive-behavioural nowadays to illustrate that problem reduction involves a wide variety of modalities.

The stages followed in cognitive-behaviour therapy are:

1. *Engagement.* The client's expectations of help are explored in a leisurely fashion, conveying the message that there is time to listen and that the worker cares. The use of open questions allows the person to talk freely.
2. *Problem focus.* Having identified some problems that could be targeted for exploration, the worker asks, 'Which problems do you most want help with?', that is prioritises.

3. *Problem assessment*. Here one specific example is examined in detail. The client is asked to describe an event, his/her underlying assumptions or inferences from it, his/her feelings, thoughts and behaviours towards the event, and 'In what ways would you like to feel, think and behave differently than you do now?', that is, goals.
4. *Teach cognitive principles* and practices of the therapy and get the person to look at his/her own thoughts; for example, teach the client to spot when he/she uses the words 'should' and 'ought', 'I should (not) have done that' or 'I ought to feel guilty' and so on.
5. *Dispute and challenge* these target assumptions.
6. *Encourage the client's self-disputing* through the use of questions. For instance, 'What evidence do you have? Is there another way of looking at this? Are your thoughts logical?'
7. *Set behavioural homework* to carry on this process and keep a diary of distorted inferences and self-evaluations.
8. *Ending*. Teach self-therapy to maintain improvement.

Motivational interviewing

Motivational interviewing is based on the acknowledged interrelationship between thought and action. It has been the subject of much analysis in working with addictive behaviour, especially alcohol addiction, and has also been used in criminal justice work. Behavioural therapies replaced counselling and alcohol education as a way of responding to addictive behaviour. Early work used Antabuse as a form of respondent conditioning. This involved administering a drug that created a nauseous reaction when alcohol was consumed. Ultimately the person addicted would associate the consumption of alcohol with nausea and would be deterred. More recently research in the area of clinical psychology led to the development of treatments based on *cognitive*-behavioural approaches. That is they linked thought process to behaviour.

The most widely used approach is based on the work of Prochaska and DiClemente (1984), where stages of change in the motivation of the person experiencing the addiction are identified and seen as forming the motivational cycle. It has been used in programmes for working with offenders addicted to alcohol. Criminal justice workers would organise their intervention around the stages of the cycle. The interventions involve work that is close to individual counselling, but also utilise some of the basic behavioural approaches outlined above.

The stages of the cycle are:

- *The precontemplative stage* where change is not necessarily desired by clients at a personal or psychological level but their circumstances cause them to consider it. Often offenders who have been sentenced for alcohol-related offences, or who identify alcohol as contributing to their offending behaviour, are at this stage.
- *The contemplation stage* involves an active structured evaluation with the worker of the pros and cons of changing and not changing. What would be the consequences of not drinking?
- *The action stage* will be a conscious and planned attempt at controlling the addictive behaviour.
- *The maintenance stage* is when the drinking is under control, but behavioural and cognitive strategies are employed to resist pressure or temptation to drink, thus avoiding the:
- *Relapse stage*, which is when there is a resumption of the addictive behaviour.

Those who are able to respond positively to the maintenance stage may move to a state where drinking is no longer seen as problematic behaviour to be consciously controlled. However many people move between stages of the cycle several times before they reach that outcome. In that there are no rules about the organisation of the cycle, people may relapse to precontemplation or contemplation.

Acknowledging this enables the worker to see such relapses as a normal part of the change cycle, and he/she will employ different forms of intervention at different stages, thus avoiding frustration and depression on the part of worker and client who might otherwise view relapses as failure. Techniques of *motivational interviewing* help the client move through the stages, which involve a series of non-confrontational practices to help people recognise for themselves the need for change by identifying the positive and negative consequences of their drinking behaviour. Uncomfortable ambivalences revealed at this stage may be resolved by acting to change the drinking pattern. In this way the desire to change has been identified by the person him or herself, which moves him/her from the precontemplative stage, although it can be revisited at different stages in the cycle.

Within motivational interviewing, other techniques include behavioural assessment methods. These involve realistic appraisal of drinking patterns, consumption level and factors that precipitate drinking. Simple versions of drink diaries or other reporting methods are used in the initial stages, but more complex recording methods can be adopted later. In discussing the use of motivational interviewing in a project with the probation service, Remington and Barron (1991) describe another specific technique – a *constructional approach to social casework*. This emphasises the need to reinforce positive motivation as well as eliminate negative behaviour. In working with the client on his/her strengths and abilities, treatment decisions are made and achievable goals identified, taking into account the function of the drinking in the person's life and trying to find other means of fulfilling that function. Remington and Barron (1991), on the basis of their research, argue that the general principles of this composite approach are relevant to a whole range of what they call 'appetite' problems, which include gambling, eating disorders, sex-related offending and the use of illegal drugs.

Apart from the positive outcomes of such approaches outlined in evaluations, a method (or collection of methods) that focuses on both the behaviour and the person's understanding of the behaviour gives some responsibility to the individual for wanting to change. Also important in making choices is an understanding of the effects of that change, both positive and negative. In this way, the individual is participating throughout the process, and can make informed choices about his/her participation, rather than having to conform to a set of behaviours imposed by the worker. Because the past is not seen as important, nor is the 'why', that is, the 'cause' of the problem pursued, some have argued that structured behavioural approaches go some way to user/client participation. The approaches are also seen to be less oppressive because labelling is discouraged and accountability is made more evident (Milner and O'Byrne, 2002).

Forrester and colleagues (2008), drawing on a large and rapidly growing literature on the effectiveness of motivational interviewing and on their own research, suggest that the client-centred values of motivational interviewing appear consistent with those of social work. They therefore suggest there are theoretical and empirical reasons for believing that it may be an appropriate approach for use by child and family social workers with parents who have alcohol-related problems, an area of work which, according to their research, social workers found very difficult.

Pro-social modelling

Another application of cognitive-behavioural approaches was developed by Trotter (2006) using the results of evaluative research into working with involuntary clients. Involuntary clients are those who either have not chosen to receive services, or have been court-mandated to receive services. Such clients challenge workers, who have the dual responsibility of legal duty or surveillance role and a commitment to helping and/or problem solving. Trotter suggests that with this group of clients a combination of accurate role clarification, working with problems and goals that are defined by the client, and modelling and reinforcing pro-social values have been found to be effective. For example, he found, in research into the work of probation officers in Australia with offenders, that using a pro-social modelling approach reduced their offending behaviour.

Pro-social modelling draws on aspects of cognitive-behaviour therapy that focus on thought patterns and changing distorted thinking. Trotter suggests that people are influenced by behaviour that is modelled by others and by positive and negative reinforcement of their own behaviour. Pro-social behaviour is developed by exposure to pro-social role models, and reinforcing and rewarding pro-social behaviour. As was said earlier in the chapter, an important factor is the nature of the rewards, the timing of the rewards and the consistency of the rewards.

In working with involuntary clients Trotter suggests that the worker has to:

- identify pro-social comments and behaviour;
- reward these with praise;
- present him or herself as a pro-social model – by demonstrating respect and self-revelation;
- challenge anti-social or pro-criminal behaviour and attitudes.

It is apparent that in this work the worker–client relationship is crucial. Trotter acknowledges that in his training courses workers often claim that they already operate in this way. However it is suggested that without proper training and without being aware of the theoretical background and need for consistency, social workers might apply some of these aspects erratically and might end up reinforcing the wrong behaviour. Trotter recognises that there are dilemmas connected to the use of power in relationships, but he asserts that, from his research and training courses, a careful and thoughtful approach can be achieved.

Overview for understanding behavioural approaches

- *The theoretical base* for behavioural approaches is learning theory, which includes respondent and operant conditioning, observational and cognitive learning.
- *Problems* that respond well to this approach include phobias, habits, anxiety, depression and obsessive-compulsive disorders (perhaps with drug treatment in tandem). Also, behavioural deficits, such as social skills, are treated through behavioural regimes.
- *Goals* are specific, observable (or self-reported in the case of something like a sexual difficulty). Goals must be stated in behavioural terms.
- *The client's role*. The person helps to measure the baseline behaviour, its frequency, intensity, duration and the context within which it occurs (see Sheldon, 1983). Diaries and other records may be kept. The client's view of what is a reward for him/her is vital, as are their goals for change. The person usually must be motivated or helped to be motivated. Where a child is the client, the carer or other change agent needs to be motivated.
- *The worker's role* is to help with the behavioural assessment and to mobilise any necessary resources. A contract may be drawn up. Strategies must be capable of being evaluated and measured for effectiveness. A concerned, genuine and hopeful relationship is necessary, if not sufficient, for change. The worker is active, sometimes directive and challenging, and an educator.
- *Techniques* include systematic desensitisation, extinction procedures and positive reinforcement, teaching self-control and thought-stopping techniques, motivating through positive construction, disputing irrational thoughts and giving information to other agents such as teachers, parents and colleagues involved in the programme.

Critique

Early critiques highlight some of the ethical problems raised in connection with using behaviourist approaches. At an early stage Jehu (1967) pointed out that to encourage people to behave in certain ways, or to attempt to extinguish behaviour that is deemed to be inappropriate or maladaptive, presents many dilemmas. The debate about 'normalisation' in work with people with learning difficulties highlights some of these (Wolfensberger, 1983). It is assumed that there are 'normal' ways of behaving, which are common to us all and should be used as some sort of yardstick for deciding whether someone is ready to live in the community. Whatever group of people we are working with, definitions of 'normal' must reflect the wide variety of behaviours demonstrated by those of us who are not subject to social work intervention. Otherwise, social workers are at risk of abusing their power and influence, and of setting inappropriate standards.

The alternative term for normalisation – age-appropriate behaviour – begs all sorts of questions about what is 'appropriate'. Such definitions must reflect differences based on, for example, class, race, ethnic background and gender, as well as age itself. In terms of race and ethnicity the Department of Health (2005), while advocating behavioural approaches, has highlighted the need to improve access to culturally appropriate counselling and psychological therapies for individuals from black and minority ethnic communities. The Improving Access to Psychological Therapies (IAPT) initiative argues that there is robust evidence to show that cognitive-behavioral therapy (CBT) is an effective treatment for people suffering from anxiety and depression. However the focus in CBT is on the individual and on treating the individual, which is based on Western concepts and illness models. For people from some communities, this will be a challenge especially if they view themselves in the context of their immediate and wider family and/or in the context of their community.

However the IAPT has suggested that a 'third wave' of CBT treatments incorporate principles such as mindfulness based CBT and meditation. For example, dialectical behavior therapy (DBT) developed by Linehan (1987) in the US to treat persons with borderline personality disorder is now being used in the UK. It combines cognitive-behavioral approaches with mindful awareness largely derived from Buddhist meditative practice.

Other criticisms of CBT argue that by focusing on the individual, the larger familial, community, societal and structural issues and problems are ignored or left unspoken and unaddressed. Smith and Vanstone recognise that CBT, at the heart of the rehabilitation programme, could be seen to contribute to social justice as it aims to both protect potential future victims and reintegrate those who offend (2002, p. 818). However an alternative view is that because it could be associated with pathologising certain individuals it might actually be counter to social justice (McNeill, 2000).

Gorman (2001) critiques the prevalence of cognitive-behavioural approaches within the criminal justice system. He associates them with the impetus to find the 'magic bullet' or Holy Grail of stopping offending behaviour. The drive for a more 'effective' service has led to a managerial approach that assumes that all offending, whatever the offence, is attributable to the failure of offenders to think through their actions and about the effect of their behaviour on others. He suggests that the 'one size fits all' approach of using cognitive-behavioural approaches in groups and applying the same 'dosage' to all, that is using the same programme material, not only denies the diversity of rationales and motivations involved in offending but seriously underestimates the potential risks (see also Weaver and McNeill, 2010). It also ignores the societal 'causes of crime'.

However, social workers do have power and that they influence those they work with in all sorts of subtle ways. For some, the fact that the aim of the intervention is made explicit is more honest than the more 'therapeutic' interventions. Sheldon (2000) argues that at the political level there are always concerns about which behaviour is to be reinforced, or extinguished, but on a case-by-case basis it is usually obvious, especially when anti-social or self-destructive behaviour is being demonstrated. As has been said, the principles of client involvement and consent can act as safeguards. In working with offenders or those demonstrating addictive behaviour, it is sometimes argued that informed consent can be linked to principles of self-determination. If someone knows the consequences of continuing to offend, or continuing to abuse harmful substances, then he or she can actively choose to be involved in a behavioural approach. However, if the alternative is the threat of a custodial sentence, or continued incarceration in either a prison or a mental hospital, then it is questionable how free such choices are.

Those who support behavioural approaches have argued that because of the structured approach and the overwhelming evidence of its success (Sheldon, 2000) it would be immoral not to use these methods. Hudson and Macdonald (1986) argue that behavioural work is usually effective because it is prepared to measure what is achieved and engages clients in working on overt behaviour which they choose to change, not covert goals which the worker thinks would be 'good' for them. It could be argued that being prepared to share skills with clients, teaching them to avoid inappropriate dependence on workers, gives clients more opportunities to achieve social acceptability.

However, as with most individual approaches, the major criticism is that it focuses on the individual and holds the individual responsible for his/her behaviour and circumstances. In this way it is supporting the status quo. Although these approaches may give the individual agency, they also involve a reductionist approach that does not take into account the social and economic circumstances that contribute to the individual's behaviour. For example, in the case of Velma, below, the race and gender considerations that are part of both her history and her current circumstances are not addressed. She has to learn to 'cope' by reacting to them in a different way.

Practice focus

Velma is a 33-year-old woman of mixed parentage. She has been diagnosed as suffering from schizophrenia. She is an intelligent woman but has had limited formal education. Her turbulent childhood included episodes of abuse by her stepfather, although this was not acknowledged until she was an adult. During her adolescence she demonstrated behaviour that led to her spending a great deal of time in residential care, although she was never charged with any offences. Frequently it was stated that she was 'at risk' because she would run away from foster homes. Eventually she was confined to a secure mental hospital, having been sectioned under the Mental Health Act when she attempted arson on her mother's house.

On discharge from hospital Velma was accommodated away from her family in a semi-secure hostel. As part of her care programme she attended a day centre, was seen by a psychologist, a psychiatrist, and had a mental health social worker as well as a key worker at the hostel. It was her hope that she would be eventually given her own accommodation in the community.

However Velma was prone to outbursts of violent behaviour when she experienced frustration. This was not directed at other people but either at herself (self-harm by cutting herself) or at objects (for example she would kick doors, break windows or smash objects). On one occasion this behaviour led to her spending a night in the police cells, and Velma was aware that because of her previous history she was at risk of losing her liberty if the behaviour continued. In her work with the psychologist to identify factors that precipitated the violence they had identified that it occurred when Velma thought people were ignoring her, or she felt she was unfairly treated. The psychologist introduced Velma to ways of trying to think differently about the situations. Although her resentment was understandable she had to recognise that when she reacted angrily it was she who was punished, not others. She was encouraged to 'take time out' and control her breathing to try and stay calm in these situations.

Meanwhile, as part of her care planning approach, the hostel staff were also working with Velma to modify behaviour that was seen to be unacceptable. For example, Velma would get very attached to particular staff and want to spend time with them, getting frustrated and angry if they were not available for her. The staff, with Velma's agreement, devised a points system. She was allocated a number of points each month, and if she behaved in ways that were deemed unacceptable by the staff she would lose points. If she went below a certain threshold she would lose privileges, such as participating in social outings or being allowed to go out by herself. The aim of this was to extinguish the 'antisocial' behaviour rather than reward good behaviour.

Velma complied and overall her behaviour did improve. However at times she suggested to her social worker that she resented the fact that she thought some staff would deduct points unnecessarily, or that the definition of what was deemed to be acceptable or unacceptable differed between staff.

Conclusion

This chapter has demonstrated that behavioural approaches adopted from psychology influence social work practice in a number of ways. 'Treatment' programmes that have been developed focus on individual behaviour and attempt to solve social problems by changing behaviour. Although there is thought to be merit in the fact that the desired outcomes of intervention are transparent, and usually negotiated, it is apparent that the methods present some ethical challenges. However it may be that these challenges exist for all social work intervention.

Point for reflection

The chapter has discussed the different ways that humans learn and how this has been incorporated into ways of working to change behaviour. This raises ethical questions about who decides behaviour should change? What behaviour should be changed? Who decides what is desirable behaviour?

These questions are fundamental to all social work practice so why do you think the methods described in this chapter cause such strong reactions?

What are your reactions to the idea that you, as a social worker, can decide how someone should behave?

Putting it into practice

Behaviour modification can operate in a variety of ways – both formally and informally – so it is important that you are aware of the way that you can influence situations.

1 Thinking about Trotter's pro-social modelling, identify a piece of work that you have been involved in. Reflect on the way that you behaved with this case. You can do this by thinking about your work over time, or by focusing on one interview. How do you think that the actions that you have taken, the words that you have used or the stance that you have taken might influence the situation? Do you nod a lot in interviews, or make encouraging noises? Do you show your disapproval? Might this be reinforcing? In what other ways might you be influencing behaviour?

2 Identify a situation from your practice in which you might consider using behaviour modification techniques (or referring someone for this kind of treatment). Write down all the reasons for using such techniques and all the reasons against using them. Are there any situations in which you feel it would be totally inappropriate? Why?

Messages from research

Hettema, J., Steele, J. and Miller, W. R. (2005) 'Motivational Interviewing', *Annual Review of Clinical Psychology*, 1, pp. 91–111. This article describes a review of seventy-two trials using motivational interviewing. There is strong evidence for its effectiveness in work with alcohol problems, and promising results with a range of other problem behaviours, including, for example, dietary change, drug problems and medication adherence.

Further resources

Cigno, K. (2002) 'Cognitive-behavioural practice' in Adams, R., Dominelli, L. and Payne, M. (eds) *Social Work: themes, issues and critical debates*. Basingstoke: Palgrave Macmillan.
A useful summary of the use of cognitive-behavioural methods in practice.

Sheldon, B. (2000) 'Cognitive behavioural methods in social care: a look at the evidence', in Stepney, P. and Ford, D. (eds) *Social Work Models, Methods and Theories*. Lyme Regis: Russell House.
This chapter argues, on the basis of research evidence, for the use of behavioural methods in social care.

Trotter, C. (2006) *Working with Involuntary Clients*, 2nd edn. London: Sage.
This book describes Trotter's research within the criminal justice system in Australia, but it gives some useful background discussion of the principles of behavioural methods and the approach can be transferred to work with other user groups.

The NHS initiative Improving Access to Psychological Therapies includes a section on working with CBT http://www.iapt.nhs.uk/?s=CBT.
The best practice guide for Psychological Wellbeing Practitioners (2010) can be accessed here.

The website for the Association of Psychological Therapies (APT) has details of specific CBT courses http://www.apt.ac/cognitive_therapy_courses.html.

PART III

Contexts of Intervention

The third part of the text focuses on the contexts in which the various methods and interventions discussed so far may be applied. Recognising that much of what is discussed in Part II can be applied to the groups identified in the following chapters, it is also the case that social work in specific 'contexts' requires consideration for a number of reasons:

- The setting has implications for the way methods of intervention are used
- Policy developments impact on the contexts for social work and shape the way skills and methods of intervention are utilised
- Additional specific methods have evolved from different settings

Obviously not all settings or contexts are covered. There is no separate chapter on criminal justice work as the place of criminal justice social work in England is contested. However, reference has been made to working with offenders throughout the text. The other omission is working in residential settings. This is because the context of the institution impacts on social work practice in residential settings in ways that require different considerations when using social work interventions (see Smith, 2009). This is not to say the processes and methods of intervention discussed in the previous sections and in this one are not relevant – but that they are complicated by the nature and purpose of the different institutions.

CHAPTER 10

Working with children and families

Introduction

The focus of this chapter is on the family as the site of intervention. Although the needs of children are paramount in policy and practice, social work is often about working with families. Many direct referrals to social work are to do with families. Referrals for practical problems sometimes uncover difficulties rooted in unsatisfactory family relationships. Assessments for community care require workers to consider family relationships, and the dynamics of these relationships influence the outcomes of such assessments. Care arrangements for older people, people with disabilities or those with mental health problems may well have to become involved in some family work using their understanding of family dynamics and specialist interventions. Workers in the criminal justice system frequently have to assess both the influence of the family on patterns of offending, and the impact of the offending on family dynamics. Families experience loss and bereavement, or they respond to counselling or short-term work.

This chapter therefore begins with a consideration of the family in this context. However, work with children is, necessarily, a high priority in social work and the chapter therefore considers this as a specific and separate topic.

Understanding families

It is impossible to advise what is a 'conventional family'. Statistical trends indicate changing demographic patterns. For example, about a third of all households have a single person at their head; households are getting smaller because fewer people are marrying and women are having fewer children (Butler and Roberts, 2004). In addition, there is diversity among families based on differences of class, race and sexual orientation. This is now being acknowledged in policies that recognise gay and lesbian couples as potential foster and adoptive parents. It is also important to remember that not only is each family different in its composition but each family differs in the way members communicate their values and their structural relationships. This attention to diversity should be at the heart of work with families.

Diversity

Media representations of families tend to subscribe to a hegemonic view of families made up of two heterosexual parents and two children. Such ideologies also influence policy and can be oppressive to families that do not fit into this model. Those who do not conform are often perceived as deviant and in some ways in deficit. This of course ignores the fact that those families that do fit the model can be oppressive and destructive, as research into domestic violence and child abuse has illustrated.

In work with families, there is danger that workers attempt to recreate a mirror image of their own family's functioning. It is vital not to generalise about families but to try to understand: 'How does *this* family work?'

Lifecycles

Trying to understand a family is like jumping on to a moving bus: you have the disadvantage of being a temporary passenger on their journey through a stage in their life, with people leaving and joining along the way. Families go through a lifecycle and at each phase in their development the whole group has to reshuffle, while at the same time providing stability and continuity for its members. Individuals go through processes of engaging and disengaging with others within some form of family unit. As such they become part of a socially constructed unit based on some form of mutuality that is based on 'a relationship of kinship, obligation and intimacy' (White, 2002, p. 147) – a family by another name.

Such processes are made all the more demanding as each member is probably struggling with his or her individual life stages at the same time: a woman who has launched children and achieved independence may be faced with a relative who is becoming dependent. All the time, families are losing members and gaining members, making space for maybe competing needs, renegotiating the numerous patterns of relationship between people – this is why referrals often have life-cycle changes at the nub of what is going wrong.

Family patterns

According to Gorrell Barnes (1984), families can be placed at one of three possible points on a spectrum from flexibility, through rigidity to chaos. Jordan (1972) illuminatingly described families that were difficult to break free from as 'integrative', and those whose members were segregated and went their separate ways as 'centrifugal': Minuchin (1974) termed these patterns of closeness and distance 'enmeshed' and 'disengaged'. These ideas may help us to assess if a family can 'bend' with its changing membership and processes (for instance, if there is adaptability of rules when a child enters adolescence). Also, albeit that there are different cultural norms, they enable us to enquire if a family is able to regulate its boundaries and can tolerate closeness and distance, dependence and independence.

Another useful concept that helps in understanding how families act and react is to see a family as a system. As discussed in Chapter 3, a system is a set of interacting parts with a particular purpose. Families may have subsystems that comprise the marital subsystem, the children subsystem, sibling subsystem, mother–daughter and father–son subsystems, and so on. The family's relationship to outside, wider systems (the suprasystem) is as important to understand as their internal dynamics. For example, suprasystems cannot be ignored when working with black families. The family is an open system in transformation, constantly changing in relation to internal and external forces. Occasionally families 'get stuck', maybe as the result of coping with their own internal crises or because the agencies, with which they interact, overreact. When this happens, solutions become part of a problem spiral. For example, services are sometimes dependent on someone being given a label, and the rise in the diagnosis of Attention Deficit Hyperactivity Disorder (ADHD) among children in families that are having difficulties coping might be the result of such a phenomenon.

Understanding the way the wider context of families can impact on them and the ways that families experience this is also important. Methods can be used to chart family relationships as part of an assessment, formal or informal, but can also form part of work with families.

Networks

Networks are particularly useful when working with families and most useful when considering families as a personal social network: one that comprises those with special and emotional significance. Hill (2002) points out that it is these networks of relatives, friends and neighbours to whom people with problems often turn. It is part of the social work task in family work to identify how far these networks have contributed to the need or problem. However, an understanding of the structures and processes in a person's or family's network also helps in assessing to what extent they can facilitate or hamper resolution of the need or problem. Hill (2002) suggests that there are ways of classifying networks by observing and documenting interactions between network members. These may be members of a family, or could include others with whom family members interact. Hence the factors to consider include:

- content
- degrees of intimacy
- frequency of contact
- directedness
- durability
- intensity. (Hill, 2002, p. 238)

An important aspect of using these categories is that there are no prior assumptions about how the network should be, but it becomes an important tool to document how things are for particular families. So plotting a network helps avoid the stereotyping of, for example, Asian families as being 'close'. It also helps to identify if families are being socially excluded because of factors such as systematic racism. In that networks can be inclusive, they can also help identify pressures and losses that, for example, asylum seekers might experience because they are separated from their families of origin.

The most frequent representation of a network is in some form of diagram. This helps workers process a great deal of information and can also be a tool that is developed interactively with the individual or family. Hill (2002, p. 244) identifies six main types of diagram:

- *The ecomap, ecogram or star diagram* where a key person is put in the centre and others are represented and connected to the key person.
- *Concentric circles* where people are placed at different distances from the central person to represent geographical or emotional closeness.
- *Genogram or family tree* depicts relationship patterns and events over generations. Births, deaths, divorce, crises and other significant life events can be recorded briefly and several pages of social history can be condensed into a diagram.

Typical symbols used in a genogram are shown in Figure 10.1. Figure 10.2 illustrates a family whose eldest son, aged 14, has committed offences. He has been brought up mainly by his mother, who is now widowed. The boy has a brother aged 10 and a sister aged 8. Prior to their father dying, the children's parents were separated. The maternal grandfather died before the grandchildren were born, though his divorced wife, the maternal grandmother, is still alive.

As with other diagrams, genograms can become a useful talking point for families who, while they are helping the worker to complete them, begin to uncover their family's unwritten rules, myths, secrets and taboos. This map of family relationships can also reveal how patterns might get repeated across generations. Thus, the family represented in Figure 10.2 had marital breakdown, death

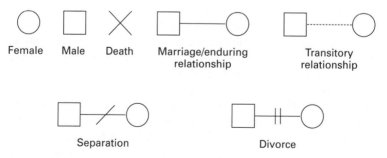

| Female | Male | Death | Marriage/enduring relationship | Transitory relationship |

| Separation | Divorce |

Figure 10.1 Genogram symbols

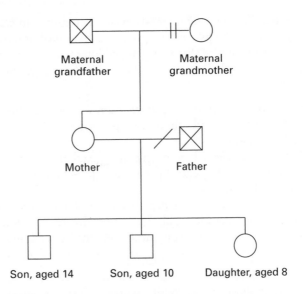

Figure 10.2 Illustrative genogram

and children reared single-handedly by their mother as repetitive themes.

Life space representation portrays key locations in an individual's life space with indications of the people and activities relevant to each. This can sometimes be drawn as a life 'snake' where the snake bends at significant points and these are named or illustrated.

Life course changes involve a sequence of houses to show changes in locality and household composition.

Matrices consist of tables listing people, their interactions, importance, function and so on, described in words rather than symbols.

These diagrams can be interactive and/or retrospective, giving opportunities for the individuals and families to personalise them (Hill, 2002). The ultimate in dynamic diagrams is family sculpting, where one member of the family places others in positions and poses to reflect the closeness of their relationship.

Often the use of such tools helps us to view the family as a small organisation (but with a shared history and future). We may see that it has a hierarchy, communication systems, values, controls, decision making, conflict resolution, norms of behaviour and ways of coping with change. Just like an organisation, a family has an invisible set of rules for how people interact with each other and how homeostasis (stability) is maintained. In order to protect themselves families develop ways of managing interactions between themselves and with outsiders. Sometimes, as has been said, these sequences and habits get in the way of moving on.

Possibly, it is only when we join an organisation that we learn how it really works. The same is true of families. As workers, it is only if we achieve an alliance (throughout the process, not just at the beginning) together with an attitude that they are 'OK', will we ever have any inkling of what is going on.

However, this is not the same as saying that we approve of everything they do. Numerous child abuse enquiries have reminded us of the need to be alert to risk of abuse. There is a tension in practice between providing support when families ask for it and the possibility of compulsory intervention (Waterhouse and McGhee, 2002). Often families might be deterred from seeking help if workers are only going to concentrate on possible abuse. Working with families requires taking time to listen to every member's point of view, being courteous, not taking sides and not confronting people with what you see as the 'truth' of their difficulties. This is more likely to encourage discussion and sharing in which the worker is free to engage and disengage when the need arises. However, workers should not shirk from their responsibility to protect children, and others, in family situations: they have to be both sceptical and compassionate.

Working with families

Work with families was originally 'family casework' (Jordan, 1972). In this model the focus was on the relationship within families. This approach developed into a 'family therapy' approach, which is used when the whole family is the client and the target for change. When one or more family members are having difficulties, this is thought to be a cause and a consequence of interaction. People affect and are affected by one another, and so it is necessary to see how people get along with each other and, more fundamentally, how the family solves its problems. This can be an important part of the assessment process.

Strategies for change that are called 'marital and family therapy' and which draw on either psychoanalytic practice or systems theory are employed and can help families and couples to draw on their own problem solving solutions and strengths. The ideas incorporated into this approach can be used practically and in a range of settings (Treacher and Carpenter, 1984) and there is evidence that family therapy is a promising treatment approach for many child and adolescent problems (Vetere, 1999, p. 145).

There are at least four theoretical viewpoints in family therapy (for more detail of these see Coulshed and Orme, 2006):

- psychoanalytic models
- structural models
- strategic models
- behavioural models

Response to criticisms

Family therapists who base their practice on systemic thinking suggest that while some events can be described in a linear, cause and effect way (that A causes B which has no feedback effect on A), this does not account for complex human interactions. To take one situation: can it be said that a husband drinks because his wife gets depressed without considering that both are involved in the sequence? Another valid explanation could be that his drinking causes the depression. Seeing events in this 'whole' or systems way reveals that each person is part of a circular system of action and reaction, which can begin and end at any point, and therefore there is little point in asking, 'Who started it?' However, one big problem with this circular view of events is that it ignores the unequal distribution of power. Where power is an obvious factor, such as the use of violence in marriage, in the main, against women, this idea of complementarity, that behaviours fit together, is questionable.

The assumption of worker expertise and the potential to 'cure' or 'solve' family problems has been critiqued in social work. As discussed in Chapter 2, constructivist approaches to social work place less emphasis on a simple definition of truth but try to elicit different understandings and experiences of problems. Circular questioning derived from family therapy can help with this. It involves asking each person in the family (or situation) to give their perspective and/or what they think is the perspective of others in the situation: for example asking a father 'when your son has a tantrum how do you think your wife feels?' Family therapy is also changing to respond to constructivist approaches and has developed techniques to help separate the person from the problem (Vetere, 1999), and to help families create positive affirming narratives about themselves that emphasise resilience rather than 'healing' (White, 2002).

There have been concerns that working with families as systems can both reinforce stereotypical gender roles. Developments in feminist approaches to social work (Featherstone, 1997; Milner, 2001) provide both a critique of family work and a framework for working with women and with significant others in their lives. Perspectives are provided on working with men developed by women (Cavanagh and Cree, 1996; Orme *et al.*, 2000) and men (Christie, 2001; Scourfield and Coffey, 2002). These approaches use a 'gender lens' and give different perspectives on, for example, the way gender-patterning contributes to the family's problems (White, 2002, p. 151). In addition, in that it questions accepted models of family functioning, it can help challenge those that ignore diversity in family structure or are imbued with heterosexist assumptions and, as has been said, incorporate oppressive assumptions about racial differences.

Family violence

Before going on to discuss other frameworks for intervening in families, it is important to spend time considering the implications of family violence for working with families. This includes both domestic violence and child protection. This section focuses on domestic violence, and its implications for children. Later in the chapter there is specific discussion of child protection.

Domestic violence

In recognising that abuse takes many forms (physical, sexual and emotional) Mullender (1996) is clear that it is physical abuse, or the anticipation of it, that keeps all other forms of abuse in place, and that the aim of such physical abuse is power and control of men over women. When considering contraindications for working with families, it seems obvious to make links between the position of women and the need to protect children from the various forms of abuse. However, the situation is more complicated than this. Children need to be protected from abuse by men, but they are also subject to abuse by women (see Wise, 1990 and Featherstone, 1997 and 2006b for discussion of the implications of this for practice). Also, studies have shown that children are witnesses to, or are aware of, the violence between their parents, and this has adverse affects, which are manifested in many different ways (Mullender and Morley, 1994). To make these claims is not to blame women for their failure to protect children, but to highlight that before any work with families is contemplated, workers need to be clear that they are not colluding with, or contributing to, abuse of women and/or children. In all work with families and couples, there has to be awareness that symptoms of abuse, or direct revelations of abuse, may be an outcome. Workers should be prepared to face such revelations, and to realise that they have implications for the way they work with families.

Mullender's research also suggests there are preconditions for family work and/or work with couples. These are:

1. The offender has accepted full responsibility for his violent behaviour and has made concerted efforts to change that behaviour.
2. The victim is clearly able to protect herself, measured by her understanding and willingness to assume responsibility for her protection.
3. The potential for future abuse is minimal (there is never a guarantee).
4. The degree of intimidation and fear felt by the victim is significantly reduced, so as not to interfere with open discussion of marital issues. Make sure she does not think the issues she raises during the session will be used as an excuse by her husband to assault her after the session.
5. The goals of the couple are mutually agreed upon and couple work is entered into freely by both partners. Make sure he has not instructed her to remain silent on contentious issues.
(Quoted in Mullender, 1996, p. 179)

This is not to say that all work should be abandoned if there are obvious signals, or even suspicions, that abuse has taken, or is taking, place. There is growing evidence of effective work with men in situations where domestic violence has been perpetrated (Day *et al.*, 2009). Mullender's position is that only when the conditions can be met should decisions be made about working with families and couples.

Working with couples

In marital or couples work, the theoretical viewpoints are similar to those in family work, in that there are psychoanalytic, structural, strategic and behavioural forms of work, usually based on systems thinking. The opportunities for such work in statutory services are limited by policy changes that mean that the emphasis in family work should be on children. However, there are situations where couple work is both helpful and necessary.

Having said that, it is important to remember that working with couples can include various arrangements for partnership that do not have to involve either legal or religious marriage ceremonies. Different partnerships and expectation of partnerships based on ethnicity, race, religion and sexual orientation have to be recognised from the outset, as is the acceptance that no partnership or relationship is immune from problems. Nor is all couple work about keeping couples together. Whether the goal is enriching the relationship or freeing the couple from it, it is the dynamic of the couple relationship, and the emotional commitment to being a couple, which are the focus of the intervention.

Although work is usually conjoint (with both partners) there is no objection to seeing only one partner. Also, as was indicated in the discussions about domestic violence, there are some situations when to insist on conjoint work might put the woman and/or the children at risk, and would be totally inappropriate (Hester and Radford, 1996).

Many of the underlying problems for couples, whatever their composition or legal status, are about intimacy and distance, sameness and difference, or how each person gets their needs met in the relationship.

Framework for understanding family and couples work

- *The theoretical base* is systems theory used in combination with psychodynamic, structural, strategic and behavioural ideas.
- *Problems* are those of family transactions; family problem solving patterns and communications that become blocked, distorted or displaced through one member.
- *Goals* are minimal, often aimed at changing overt behaviour, though some methods aim at insight as well. The family is

helped to choose limited, specific goals, usually within a brief timeframe. Workers aim to join the family or couple, inasmuch as they offer support while attempts are made at restructuring relationship patterns and behavioural sequences.

- *The client's role.* In this approach, the couple or the family is the client. They may also be the target for change, and the team that works alongside the therapeutic team to change transactional patterns within or outside their system.
- *The worker's role.* There may be two workers as co-therapists or a therapeutic team. Work with external systems could be just as important, especially when numerous agencies are involved who unwittingly mirror family dynamics. It is vital to sustain the couple's or the family's attempt at problem solving; to not take sides or allocate blame; not to perpetuate power inequalities but to raise awareness of these and to offer a positive redefinition of their difficulties to help those who have become stuck trying 'more of the same'.
- *Techniques* are numerous. Joining and restructuring operations include tracking communications and themes about family life. Intensity around the specific problem might be necessary in order to break out of 'redundant' problem solving routines. Observation is as important as listening, so that process and content, how the family behave and what is said, are clues to helping. Finally it is necessary to be careful not to undermine the family's competence but to confirm their strengths.

Families and children

So far this chapter has deliberately not concentrated on work with children in families. There is a growing amount of specialist litera-ture that is particularly helpful in these areas. This literature draws on research to evaluate the effectiveness of family work (Hill, 1999); gives overviews and discussion of practice initiatives with families (Bell and Wilson, 2002); and children (Brandon *et al.*, 1998; Colton *et al.*, 2001). Butler and Roberts (2004) provide very practical workbook approaches to working with children and families.

Developments that have taken place in working with families that are not heavily 'therapeutic' draw upon the notion of the family as a system and work with the potential within the family. These developments are part of wider changes that have been taking place in work with families and children. Such changes are a reaction to the number of enquiries into the role of social work in cases of child abuse and what was seen as an increasing focus on the 'deficit' notion of families. Intervention in families always has to balance the needs of families with protection of children which tends to dominate policy and practice.

For example, an overview of twenty pieces of research in 1995 (Department of Health, 1995) concluded that, overall, when child protection investigations take place little account is taken of the context; parents were generally left feeling alienated and angered; and a disproportionate amount of resources were being taken up in investigation, which took away resources from prevention and support. Overall, the principles of partnership that had been enshrined in the 1989 Children Act were not operating (Frost *et al.*, 2003, p. 26). Calls for refocusing (DoH, 1996) were supported by organisations such as family rights groups which argued for involvement and empowerment of families in the decision-making processes. However, these two things are not synonymous. Research into child protection procedures had indicated that a procedural approach to involving families in formal meetings could be just as exclusionary as no involvement at all (Department for Education, 2010). This is supported by the final report of the Munro review (Department for Education, 2011) which concludes that services are so standardised that they do not provide the required range of responses to the variety of need that is presented in child protection cases.

Two different initiatives highlight the possibility of changing approaches within statutory services to ensure families are empowered and supported and their needs are met.

Family group conferences

Based on original projects in New Zealand that had been initiated by Maori groups, the introduction of Family Group Conferences in England were an attempt to reduce the role of the state and re-emphasise the responsibilities of families and the wider community for care of their children (Lupton, 1998). The model, which was used in child welfare and youth justice, gave families support for their decision making. There was collaboration with families rather than direction. The principles were that the social worker attended a family group conference at the beginning stages to give information, but then withdrew to allow the family to discuss their 'problems' in private and develop a family plan.

The conference itself is convened by an independent coordinator and in the third stage the coordinator joins the family to be informed of the plan. Lupton's research (1998) is cautious in concluding exactly how empowering such an approach can be. For example, it is the social worker and not the family who decides there should be a conference, and there is no guarantee that resources will be made available.

In Scotland, the introduction of Family Group Conferences was not such a different way of working as Children's Panels had worked with the whole family over a number of years. The Changing Lives Report (Scottish Executive, 2006a) highlights the success of Family Group Conferencing in the area of child protection. It references international evidence that a family-centred and structured decision-making process has produced good results in diverting children from the child protection system, reducing offending behaviour and preventing some children being accommodated away from home. Children 1st (a Scottish voluntary organisation) worked with twelve Scottish local authorities to implement the approach. In one Scottish council of 30 children, rated as being medium to high risk of becoming accommodated, 26 remained in kinship care nine months after a family group conference (Scottish Executive, 2006a, p. 50). These findings are in line with projects in other parts of the UK (Brown, 2003) that found family group conferences were being used to divert families away from formal child protection procedures.

Such initiatives indicate the need to think differently about ways of working with children and families, based on principles of partnership rather than treatment. However, ten years after their introduction, Brown (2003) concludes that in the UK the role that family group conferences appear to play, within the overall number of decisions being taken about children's lives and futures, remains relatively small and the approach remains on the margins of practice. There is no real change in philosophy or practice: families do not have the right to ask for a family group conference and rely upon their social worker to suggest it.

Family support

Another initiative that attempts to move the focus from child protection to more supportive interventions is 'family support'. Initially defined as 'any activity or facility ... aimed at providing advice and support to parents to help them bringing up their children' (Audit Report Commission, 1994, p. 39), this should involve support that has no stigma attached. It should be available across the board and accessible to all who need it (Frost *et al.*, 2003, p. 5). Four levels of support reflect services that should be available to all:

- *Level One*: Projects and services such as SureStart. That is centres that bring all the different support agencies together to offer a range of services to meet the needs of all children and families – all in one place.
- *Level Two*: Targeted services addressing expressed need that is individually family-focused and might include casework or family therapy.
- *Level Three*: Where there are more severe problems of child-care/child protection, more intense services might be made available, for example, support for families where parents have drug and/or alcohol problems.
- *Level Four:* Rehabilitation services which support the return to families of those who have been looked after.

Some were suspicious of the motives of the government policy that introduced family support (Featherstone, 2006a) and universal provisions of schemes such as SureStart are under threat from changes in policy. Others such as Holman (1998), whose work with families has been community-based, argued for a revision of the organisation of services that would be family-focused. He wanted both a neighbourhood approach and a 'facility' approach – that is, day care and family centres should be provided in all communities. Alternatively, Waterhouse and McGhee (2002) suggest that partnerships need to be developed at a variety of levels: with other professions, with parents and children, and with residential care.

Family support systems based on these ideas might be able to be more responsive to the changing needs of families and the challenges that impact on family dynamics and functioning, by, for example, substance abuse (Forrester *et al.*, 2008) and HIV (Cree and Sidhva, 2011).

Discussions about family support illustrate that childcare policy and practice is an area that is subject to political agendas. Over the last decade there have been developments such as the establishment of the Children's Workforce Development Council (CWDC) in England to improve the quality and status of the children's services' workforce and children's commissioners throughout the UK to promote and protect the rights and welfare of children and young people. These reflect increasing attention to children and young people as citizens for whom the state has a responsibility beyond that of protection. However, despite those initiatives, there is still a sense that much policy and practice is driven by reaction to child abuse cases and administrative systems to identify and protect vulnerable children as the Munro review has identified (DfE, 2010; 2011).

Child protection

Child protection is a crucial area of social work, and one of the most complex. This is because the consequences of a mishandled child-abuse enquiry can be injury (both physical and emotional) and/or child death. It is therefore understandable that research and policy focuses on good practice to try and prevent abuse and protect children. The Munro Review (DfE, 2011) has questioned how the system has evolved to be so focused on procedures and guidance. The interim report attempted to redirect emphasis on to the importance of the social work skills in working with children and families. The conclusions indicated the need for integration of both policy and practice and a focus on both children and families, while the final report recommended infrastructures to support effective child and family social work that can implement evidence-based ways of working with children and families. The Munro Review definition of good social work practice includes both:

- forming a relationship with the child and family, and
- using professional reasoning to judge how best to work with parents. (DfE, 2010)

Skills for work with children generally, and in the area of child protection specifically, have been discussed already in this text. Discussion of approaches that involved counselling in Chapter 6 explains the relevance of attachment theory in understanding relationships in childhood and beyond. In Chapter 4, we looked at the specifics of communicating with children and in Chapter 3 the discussion of assessment of risk drew on work specifically in the area of child protection, as did Chapter 5, when discussing the necessity for reflection and review.

As well as taking a critical reflective approach to their practice, social workers should also heed the voices of children and young people. The CWDC summarises the key characteristics that children and young people look for in a social worker. These are:

- willingness to listen and show empathy, reliability, taking action, respecting confidences, and viewing the child or young person as a whole person and not overly identifying a child with a particular problem, and
- ability to communicate with children of varying abilities and address the emotional needs of children at key points in their lives. (DfE, 2010, p. 42)

Such a summary hints at the scale of relevant skills and knowledge required for working in the area of child protection. In particular, strengths-based and solution-focused work discussed in Chapter 8 and relationship-based therapy are also seen to be important.

Resilience

Specific strengths-based approaches relating to children include work on resilience (see for example, Daniel and Wassell, 2002). Resilience refers to the qualities that cushion a vulnerable child from the worst effects of adversity and that may help a 'child or young person to cope, survive and even thrive in the face of great hurt and disadvantage' (Gilligan, 1998). While much of the work on resilience has been undertaken in the area of looked-after children, the findings can be transferred to other work with children and young people. The aim of good practice, supported by the appropriate policies, is to find ways to boost a child's resilience: his or her positive ways of coping. Even though it might not be possible to protect children from negative experiences, increasing resilience should enhance the likelihood of better long-term outcomes. It is achieved by providing strong supportive relationships. Helping to increase self-esteem and facilitating advocacy in the policies and services that relate to them is also vital for children and young people whatever their background or experience. Hence the sustaining practices of social work intervention are vital in working with families and children to get the most positive outcomes.

Conclusion

This chapter has explored social work practice in the context of working with families and children. Work with families is relevant in every aspect of social work practice but the chapter draws particular attention to how changes in policy and practice influence practice with children and families. The chapter therefore illustrates how, in this policy context, many of the skills and methods of intervention discussed in this text are relevant to working with families and children. While acknowledging child protection as an important area, the chapter has sought to highlight that children should be seen as more than 'victims of abuse' and positive intervention with children and families is vital. Moves to a more holistic approach that treats children as citizens can lead to better outcomes for both children and families.

Practice focus

Sue, 13, had not been to school for a year. The school social worker had never seen her as Sue refused to come downstairs during home visits. A psychiatric assessment was planned, but the family, which included three older sisters who had all left home, agreed instead to work as a group. Co-workers, one male and one female, from an area social services team saw the family at home in the evenings on four occasions. Prior to contact, the workers hypothesised from the family lifecycle stage and the family tree that Sue might be struggling with adolescent challenges while her parents faced reforming as a couple, preparing for the prospect of their last child leaving home.

The workers knew from the school social worker that father was a long-distance lorry driver, who had never been interviewed, and that mother and daughter were very close. There was some suggestion of marital violence throughout the marriage, plus some strict disciplining of the three other sisters. The workers hypothesised that the women needed to ally themselves against the father's physical power. Also, when men are temporarily absent from the family and return at intervals from their jobs, this increases strain on the couple, who have continually to renegotiate space, decision making and roles.

On each visit, timed to coincide with the father's trips home, the workers often had to wait for him to arrive. Though there was some pressure to begin without him, this was resisted because this would have been no different from previous problem solving, which had not produced change. The workers had to demonstrate to the family that they were 'with them', but at the same time objectively trying to help them sort out Sue's non-attendance at school. So the meetings were kept informal until father arrived.

Bringing the whole family together seemed to help unblock communications. Father was a large-built man, quite intimidating looking but the workers treated him as if he were cooperative. Although Sue never spoke, she listened intently as her father was confronted with his over-zealous disciplining. He asserted he had never hit Sue. He looked astonished when his wife said that she intended leaving him once Sue had left school, but that she would expect Sue to accompany her. She indicated that she planned to get a full-time job and establish her independence.

The use of circular questioning revealed different viewpoints, introducing new information about how each party saw relationships in the family, in regard to the specific problem. For example, the workers asked, 'When your mother rows with your father, what does Sue do?' and, 'When your mother leaves home, who will be most, and who will be least, upset?'

The workers interpretation was that Sue was sacrificing her growing up in order to keep the family together. They thought the sessions provided a channel for the family talking about something that had been simmering for some time but that all were afraid to confront. It took the focus away from Sue as the 'problem child'.

Point for reflection

Read the above practice example that incorporates many points discussed in this chapter. Note your reaction to the situation. Do you think the workers 'interpretation' of what was going on was appropriate? What other explanations might there be? Did the opportunities offered meet the needs of everyone? What other approaches might have been taken?

Putting it into practice

This chapter has indicated that there are many ways of working with families and many tools to help that work. It is useful to practise some of these before using them with families in distress.

1 Drawing a family: in the first instance practise using the symbols to denote the different people in the 'family'.

2 Drawing a network: choose a family with whom you are working. Using one of the methods for depicting families described in this chapter draw a diagram representation of this family as you see their relationships. Think about why you are putting different people in different places – on what basis are you doing this? What does this say about the way you see the family 'functioning'?

3 Getting feedback: think about sharing this technique with the family (or one member of the family) to help understand their perception. It is important that you only do this if it makes sense in the context of the work you are doing. It is not appropriate to practise on families just for the sake of it. If you are able to use the exercise with a family, or family member, then compare what they have drawn with your own drawing and look at the points of difference, and how this might help you understand better what is happening in the family.

Further resources

Butler, I. and Roberts, G. (2004) *Social Work with Children and Families*. London: Jessica Kingsley.
This text is focused on the practicalities of working with families, but with exercises and activities to help think more widely about the implications of working with children and families.

Featherstone, B. (2004) *Family Life and Support: a feminist analysis*. Basingstoke: Palgrave.
Using a feminist analysis, this text looks at family roles and relationships and the meaning of family support.

Hill, M. (ed.) (1999) *Effective Ways of Working with Children and their Families*. London: Jessica Kingsley.
A useful edited text that draws together results from research to describe effective ways of working with children and families.

There is a great deal of research published in the area of working with children. Rather than detail specific studies reference is given to resources which provide overviews of research.

The Research in Practice website http://www.rip.org.uk/index.php/research-evidence: provides an overview of evidence relating to good practice in working with children and families.

Messages from Research http://www.dartington.org.uk/book/child-protection-messages-research. This provides an overview of research in the area of child protection with a summary of the implications for policy and practice.

The website for the Munro Review http://www.education.gov.uk/munroreview/ gives the details of the context and process of the review and access to all the reports.

The Centre for Excellence and Outcomes in Children and Young People's Services (c4eo) website http://www.c4eo.org.uk/ provides information about excellence in local practice and national research and data about 'what works'.

Working with adults

Introduction

Changes in the way that social work is organised to work with adults began with the community care reforms of the 1990s and continue in the 21st century. Community care and care management introduced philosophies for the provision of services built on notions of the market into care. This altered practice for those involved in delivering those services.

Criminal justice social work was excluded from these arrangements but did not escape reform. In England and Wales a separate service, the National Offender Management Service (NOMS) replaced the probation service and training does not necessarily rely on social work principles. In England, there is a continuing debate about whether offenders should be part of a social work service (Smith, 2005). In Scotland, despite a change in terminology to 'community justice' the services remain based on social work skills and values (McNeill and Whyte, 2007) and as such are given due attention in the 21st Review of Social Work in Scotland (McNeill *et al.*, 2005). This constitutes a major topic in its own right, which will not be part of this chapter, although at other points in the book reference has been made to the use of social work methods in criminal justice settings.

Community care and care management

The key components of community care, as interpreted by the policy initiatives that introduced it, are:

• services that respond flexibly and sensitively to the needs of individuals and their carers;
• services that allow a range of options for consumers;
• services that intervene no more than is necessary to foster independence;
• services that concentrate on those with the greatest need.
  (DoH, 1989a, para. 1.10, p. 5)

The introduction of the role of 'care manager' challenged social work practice with adults. The title is now used interchangeably with 'social worker' but the distinctions are blurred. Is the work of a care manager and a social worker synonymous? What does care management involve? The guidelines that accompanied the original legislation suggested it is not necessary to be a qualified social worker to be a care manager. The introduction of registration of social workers in 2005 protected the title of social worker for those who had a professional social work qualification from an approved course of social work training. It did not however define what social workers did.

Care management

The care management process aims to achieve planned goals using what are familiar and central tasks in social work, namely data collection, analysis and planned intervention. These could be equated to early social work processes namely study, diagnosis and treatment. The requirement that care management involves 'The process of tailoring services to individual needs' (para. 7, *Summary of Practice Guidance*: DoH, 1991) suggests that care managers require practice skills such as interviewing, communicating, assessing, recording, counselling and mobilising resources. Care management might also be seen to draw on the values of individualisation and respect for persons (see Orme and Glastonbury, 1993, for a discussion). The use of the term 'care' management in preference to the North American term 'case' indicates a move away from the individualised approach which had been the focus of casework, to emphasis on service delivery: it is the care that is to be managed and not the case or person. These developments have been emphasised by subsequent policy innovations including direct payments and personalisation.

Care management, either as a practice or as a method of organising service delivery or a method of intervention, draws on systems theory discussed in Chapter 5 (Orme and Glastonbury, 1993). It is a practice or set of practices that involves individual workers mediating arrangements and services for individuals in need. Hence social work with adults involves systematic practice (Thompson, 2002). This means that good practice requires clear planning, defined goals and a holistic assessment. In 'managing' the delivery of services, care management deals with different parts of the service user system, with the understanding that this will impact on other parts of the system. Therefore, the provision of a care assistant might enable a service user to remain in their own home if they wish to do so. This will not only improve his or her sense of self, it will relieve pressure on the family as carers and on residential accommodation.

The separation of assessment of need from determination of the service response based on the resources that are available is now translated into a shorthand version, 'purchaser/provider split'. This division was introduced to ensure the development of a mixed economy of welfare, with a greater involvement of voluntary and independent sector agencies in the provision of facilities in the community. The aim was to provide more choice for users and carers, and to find more flexible ways of maintaining people in the community.

One consequence of the purchaser/provider split is that it is often assumed that care management equates solely with the process of assessment for the purposes of community care. However, care management is more than this. At its simplest level, it can be described as a circular process of case finding and screening – assessment – planning, monitoring and review – (and eventual closure) (Department of Health, 1991). This provides a useful 'action checklist' for practitioners of seven core tasks in arranging care for someone in need as shown in Figure 11.1.

Stages 3 onwards reflect the circular process of much social work intervention that preceded care management, and which is recognised as good practice in areas such as childcare and working with offenders. As such, it could be said that care management is a codification of the social work process, and that performance of all these tasks remains dependent upon core social work skills that include interviewing, assessment, negotiation, consultation and counselling. Seemingly new processes such as advocacy and

Stages of care management

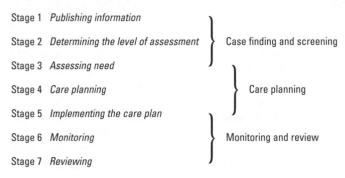

Figure 11.1 Stages of care management

working in partnership (discussed in Chapter 3) draw on many of these basic skills, but are often employed in different circumstances, or with people other than those traditionally defined as users of the social work agencies. For example, negotiating skills may be used with line managers in order to secure resources for particular users' needs, or with representatives of a voluntary agency in order to ensure that a particular need is provided for.

The original research that led to the development of care management in the UK was undertaken with older people (Challis *et al.*, 1990) and subsequent research evaluating its implementation (see for example, Postle, 2001; Postle 2002 and Gorman and Postle, 2003) also relates to the experiences of older people, or those who work with them. Care management now applies to all adult service users.

The continuing debate already alluded to is whether care management is a social work method. Horder (2002) suggests that, as it defines what social workers should do and how they should go about their work, it is a social work method. However Gorman and Postle (2003) argue that the 'reality' of care management is that it has turned social workers into brokers of services involving them in bureaucracy, paperwork and the use of computer software to undertake detailed financial assessments and issue contracts. Their research found that social workers felt deskilled because the emphasis was on management, and particularly management of risk, rather than on care. This is accompanied by a sense that 'real' social work, often described as counselling or face-to-face work, is disappearing (Postle, 2001).

Other research suggests that despite their misgivings social workers, operating as care managers, have about the same level of face-to-face contact as they did prior to the introduction of care management. Weinberg *et al.* (2003) undertook one of the few comparisons based on the actual time social workers spend with users. They found that there was, in fact, little change in the balance of activities between, for example, direct work with service users and paperwork or administration. In particular, they found that social workers have a great deal of input into answering the needs of service users and their families (Weinberg *et al.*, 2003). This is sometimes called direct work, and involves finding practical solutions to problems, a service that is valued by service users.

However, need is not always alleviated just by the provision of practical help. The sense that workers had of having less contact might be because the content and quality of direct work had changed. So, while those undertaking care management tasks might have contact with individual service users, this might be focused on highly complex assessment forms and testing out eligibility criteria. As was discussed in Chapter 2, the process of undertaking an assessment is just as important as the content, and assessment schedules can sometimes interfere with that process.

Care Programme Approach (CPA)

A well-developed system of care management for people requiring mental health services is the Care Programme Approach (CPA). This tends to be distinguished from care management because it is led by health services, as opposed to social work or social care services. As discussed in Chapter 5, the CPA was introduced in England to ensure people do not become 'lost' in systems. It focuses on the whole programme of intervention, including the management of medication.

The stages of CPA constitute an important practice guide. They ensure that the original assessment is kept firmly in view, and all those involved in the service user's system – care workers, professionals, family and friends and/or advocates – are involved in the staged reviews. Importantly, it provides the service user the opportunity to give feedback on the services they are receiving and reviews can bring about changes in any aspect of the care plan: medication, place of residence, opportunities for activity, etc.

One significant aspect of the CPA approach is that it involves inter-agency work to ensure that a range of services are accessed to provide a holistic approach to meeting the needs of service users. The other is that it is intended to involve the service user in all aspects of decision making.

This approach has implications for other changes in the way that adult services are delivered:

1. The notion of a shared assessment – incorporated into developments for a single shared assessment.
2. Person-centred planning approach – the forerunner of personalisation policies.

Single shared assessment

Central to community care arrangements is the creation of an indi-vidualised, flexible package of care, requiring workers to arrange and provide services from independent, voluntary and statutory groupings. Often such packages of care involve a number of differ-ent services/agencies, and a key responsibility of a care manager is collaboration with medical, nursing and other caring agencies (DoH, 1989a). Ideally, the care manager is the person who facili-tates and coordinates multi-professional activity designed to provide a holistic assessment. Health assessments of older people can take place at home, in a day or residential centre or in a hospi-tal setting and can involve various professionals (for instance, health visitors, occupational therapists, physiotherapists, general practitioners, district nurses and social workers).

Such assessments represent good practice, and it might be assumed that professionals would agree about categories for assess-ment from their different perspectives, but custom, practice and professional expertise mean they did not. For example difficulties in rising from a chair might be assessed:

- by a GP as arthritic hips;
- by a health visitor as a low chair;
- by a physiotherapist as poor hand function;
- by a social worker as limiting mobility and opportunities for socialising.

Because of such potential differences in approach to assessment, policy guidance was issued to require effective joint working. Single shared assessments were made a requirement for working with older people (Scottish Executive, 2000; DoH, 2000b; DoH, 2001). These directives recognised that social work assessments frequently ignored or minimised health needs, and health assessments did not address social issues. Single shared assessments are therefore designed to avoid concentrating on a single aspect of a person's situation, and to reduce the number of assessment 'events' service users and their carers have to undergo. They are expected to:

• be person-centred and needs-led
• relate to level of need
• be a process not an event

To achieve this, agencies (including local authorities, NHS services and housing departments) are required to have joint protocols and joint training. This means that a lead professional from any agency can coordinate documents, share appropriate information, coordinate all contributions and produce a single summary assessment of needs in ways that are acceptable to all professionals involved, whatever their professional setting. Assessment tools were produced to help coordinate assessments.

A single shared assessment does not decrease the number of professionals involved; the expertise from each is still required. Best practice (DoH, 2002a) dictates that the process should include local stakeholders in the assessment, including older people, service users, carers and providers. A single shared assessment should avoid the duplication of information provided by the service user and carer and ensure that no significant factors are overlooked. The differences in practice will occur in sharing information and agreement about how to respond to the needs of the individual. On addition, the service user and his/her carer will be aware of the assessment process and its results.

The guidance for local implementation of single shared assessment summarised by Parker and Bradley (2003) covers two main aspects of assessment:

• Processes for preparing for and initiating assessment. To include agreement on language, purpose and culture of the assessment.
• Processes of undertaking the assessment. To include stages for gathering and collating information and developing tools to assist this. (Parker and Bradley 2003, p. 30)

Both of these require those involved to develop shared values and joint training, and have major implications for multi-professional working. They also have to be mindful that the purpose of assessment is to put the individual at the centre of planning.

Person-centred planning

Person-centred planning was developed initially among service users with physical disabilities, and represents a move away from counselling associated with medical and tragedy models of disability (see Oliver, 1996, for discussions of models of disability). Hence while there may seem to be similarities between person-centred planning and person-centred counselling (see Chapter 6), the similarities are predominantly in the title. The medical and tragedy models of disability assumed that because individuals had an impairment they were either ill, or were grieving for the loss of not being 'able-bodied'. Such attitudes deny the personhood of people with disabilities because they focus only on their needs in a negative way and ignore the strengths that people bring to their situation.

Person-centred planning can be used with many adult users of social services and in children's services. It is usually associated with needs-led assessments and should inform good practice throughout contact with service users, including long-term contact, service provision and review.

Petch (2002, p. 226) identifies 17 aspects of person-centred planning, but these can be summarised as follows:

- Focus on the individual as unique and special, the person in his/her situation.
- At the same time recognise that some needs are universal, common to all.
- Facilitate communication and participation throughout all the processes.
- Operate in a culture of rights and entitlements.
- Make plans for monitoring and review to inform long-term goals.

As such, this approach is crucial in shared assessments and multi-professional work described below because the person can very easily become a 'case' defined by his/her problem or illness. It is vital in organisation for community care to counteract bureaucratic tendencies to categorise individuals. Person-centred planning draws on strengths-based approaches described in Chapter 8 and is, therefore, based more on the principles of justice rather than on problematic understandings of care (Orme, 2002b). It is only by recognising and responding to the circumstances of individual users that these principles can be reflected in service delivery.

Personalisation

Policies that introduced personalisation (DoH, 2008b) could be seen to be a direct development of person-centred planning, but it was the policies that introduced direct payments (Community Care (Direct Payments) Act, 1997) that had the most influence.

As stated in Chapter 3 in the development of service user involvement, there was a clear sense from some user groups that it is only when service users are given control over their own care that they can be empowered. This was interpreted in policy terms as being given the means to purchase their own care and led to the introduction of direct payments. This development had negative associations for some of the 'commodification' of care: care services are purchased as a commodity, like furniture or food. This has complicated implications for workers because the suggestion is that there is no need for social work input. The positive consequence is that direct payments allow the service user to become her/his own care manager. However, there is still a role for workers to be involved, even at a distance, because arrangements for care break down and service users' situations change and deteriorate.

Personalisation has taken the principles of direct payments even further and is seen as the goal of user participation and empowerment that user-led organisations have been striving for. Government documents throughout the UK present policies of personalisation as the ultimate in citizenship and empowerment and are intended to ensure that individual needs for independence, wellbeing, and dignity are met: 'better support, more tailored to individual choices and preferences in all care settings' (DoH, 2008b, p. 5).

In terms of social work practice, personalisation is said to involve a totally new perspective:

> This means starting with the person as an individual with strengths, preferences and aspirations and putting them at the centre of the process of identifying their needs and making choices about how and when they are supported to live their lives. (Carr, 2010, p. 3)

In terms of good social work the first part of this statement is not new – social workers have always been urged to 'start where the client (or service user) is' – to respect them and to treat them as a person in their own right (Biestek, 1957; Plant, 1973; Banks, 2006). However, what is new is the suggestion that the person should be at the centre, not only of choices, but also of service provision. The ideal of personalisation is that people get the right help at the right time and are given control. In practice it involves:

- tailoring support to people's individual needs;
- ensuring that people have access to information, advocacy and advice to make informed decisions about their care and support;
- finding new collaborative ways of working (sometimes known as co-production) that support people to actively engage in the design, delivery and evaluation of services;
- developing local partnerships to co-produce a range of services for people to choose from and opportunities for social inclusion and community development;
- developing the right leadership and organisational systems to enable staff to work in creative, person-centred ways;
- embedding early intervention, re-ablement and prevention so that people are supported early on and in a way that's right for them;
- recognising and supporting carers in their role, while enabling them to maintain a life beyond their caring responsibilities;
- ensuring all citizens have access to universal community services and resources – a total system response. (Carr, 2010, pp. 3–4)

Although hailed as a radical shift and a transformation in social care, careful consideration of the above list indicates that many of the processes and skills discussed so far in this book (e.g. communication, assessment, advocacy, partnership, solution-focused and strengths-based approaches) have to be mobilised to meet the requirements of personalisation. Underpinning the policies of personalisation is the principle that there will be allocation of personal budgets to enable service users to pay for and manage their own support services. This means that what might be called a 'whole system' approach is required, that is, it has implications for the provision of education, health provision, housing, transport – in fact all services. Therefore approaches to social work that involve whole communities, such as those discussed in Chapter 13 will also be important.

While personalisation has been welcomed by user-led organisations (ULOs) and was launched as a flagship policy that gave choice and control to service users, some commentators have raised questions about 'which users?' Barnes (2011), for example, argues that the image of 'people' in personalisation policies is gender, class and culture neutral. It does not recognise the reality and diversity of service users' situations, that is, with lives blighted by poverty, inequality, oppression and stigma, meaning they have very limited choices. Service users are often not 'the author of their own lives' (Ferguson and Woodward, 2009). She also argues that service users have to have a high level of self-knowledge and reflexivity together with management skills to operate personal budgets. While there is no reason to question that some service users have such qualities, the lack of choice and the sometimes chaotic situations in which some have to live means that their needs and circumstances will not remain stable and predictable. This may well affect their willingness to take on responsibility of constantly reviewing whether the support and help being given is enabling the achievement of objectives (Barnes, 2008, pp. 156–7). The negative consequences of the policies for Ferguson and Woodward (2009) are that risk and responsibility are transferred from the local authority to individual service users.

The suggestion that workers should work with service users in developing infrastructures for personalisation should also be treated with caution. Ferguson and Woodward (2009) suggest that for social workers and managers to impose themselves on service users who have no use for them has echoes of paternalism (2009, p. 161). They argue that where it is necessary for practitioners to work with service users, principles of partnership should prevail. Service users and carers should be afforded the same respect as other professionals involved in joint working.

Multi-professional teamwork

Multi-professional teamwork is crucial whenever we attempt to put together a rounded picture of the circumstances of people requiring care. Multi-professional teams consist of a number of different disciplines sharing their knowledge and expertise about a specific client with the objective of identifying and using those services that most effectively meet assessed needs (see DoH, 1989a). As Petch (2002) points out, community mental health teams and community disability teams provide examples of multi-professional work because they consist of workers from different agencies or professions. Arrangements might include:

- a single agency team (e.g. those based in social services but consisting of different professionals);
- a multi-agency and multi-professional team bringing together, for example, social workers, social work assistants, home care workers, community nurses, occupational therapists and housing and welfare rights specialists. (Petch, 2002)

The following skills required of individual workers, while identified some time ago, are still relevant:

- *Partnership*, the ability to engage with colleagues, allocate tasks and give feedback.
- *Negotiation*, making clear what outcomes for self and others are desired; compromise and confrontation.
- *Networking*, gathering and disseminating information, linking people and establishing mutual support groups.
- *Communicating*, writing effective reports, speaking and writing in a non-jargonised way.
- *Reframing*, offering different perspectives by placing the problem in a wider frame of reference and discussing alternative ways of seeing the problem.
- *Confronting*, assertively challenging a dominant view;
- *Flexibility*, learning from the skills of others.
- *Monitoring and evaluation*, measuring outcome and modifying methods or goals accordingly. (CCETSW/IAMHW, 1989)

Whatever kind of organisational arrangement, partnership working requires respect, openness and client-centredness if they are to make a distinctive contribution to the team. Otherwise individual workers could become either hostile or marginal figures or, chameleon-like, opt to fit in with the view of the rest. While consensus is not the goal of multi-professional working, honest dialogue can expand everyone's skills and horizons. However there has to be acceptance of the final assessment.

As Petch (2002) points out, management structures are vital. Managers have to have the respect of the team, and workers have to accept different management structures. Many of the tensions that arise amongst team members relate to the myths and stereotypes that we hold about other professions. Stereotyping can be overcome via joint training, working and peer supervision activities in multi-disciplinary teams.

Working with carers

The legislation introducing community care highlighted the need for carers to be recruited from a variety of sources, but assumed that informal carers would be predominantly family, friends and/or neighbours. There have been many criticisms of such policies because they involve subsidising statutory services by informal and unpaid labour which is often provided by women (see Orme, 2001a, for a discussion of this).

While the introduction of direct payments and personalisation have brought about changes in the way care is purchased and provided, there is still a huge army of informal carers. That care is a 'burden' is now recognised by the existence of a charter for carers and many support mechanisms. However, to express care in this way is problematic because it means that those who require care could be seen to be the burden (Morris, 1993). Nevertheless, it has to be acknowledged that informal carers are undertaking responsibilities that could/should be provided by statutory services either directly or by commissioning and paying for them from voluntary and independent sector agencies. Undertaking these responsibilities creates stress, and can also mean that those who provide that care are denied their own identity; they are seen only as the carer (Barton, 2002).

The complexities and demands of being a carer were recognised by the introduction of the Carers (Recognition and Services) Act (1995), which gave carers the right to an assessment. The implementation was patchy and even if care managers were spending time with individuals, research found that relatively small amounts of time was spent with carers (Weinberg *et al.*, 2003; Carpenter and Schneider, 2004).

Charters and other documents represent rights for carers, but fulfilling these rights is not straightforward. While it might be true that the traditional role of the social worker as the link person with the family is being fulfilled by care management (Carpenter and Schneider, 2004, p. 381), that traditional role has also been criticised for pathologising individuals and for drawing people into the welfare net unnecessarily. While there is an imperative to recognise 'service users and their carers' it has to be remembered that carers are not necessarily service users (although of course they might be: service users can also provide care), they are service providers. Because of this there is an obvious imperative that social workers, when working with carers, have to operate according to the principles of just practice. This will include:

- treading a fine line between being responsive to carers' needs and recognising the stress of caring, but not assuming that the person who is providing care either has problems or is a problem;
- recognising that, like service users, carers are not a unified group;
- responding to carers as service providers;
- balancing the rights and needs of carers with the rights and needs of service users.

Working with carers highlights that the provision of care often raises issues of competing needs between those who require care and those who provide it. This, and the need to recognise diversity of people receiving care and those providing care, is linked to notions of 'just' practice.

'Just' practice

Driven by the need to provide 'care' and to ensure that they are meeting managerial targets for time taken to provide assessments, workers can often stereotype service users by labelling and assuming they all share the same characteristics. Issues of gender (Orme, 2001a) or race (Ahmad and Atkins, 1996) influence assessments and service provision in community care and can involve two phenomena:

1. Workers operate according to categories that have been developed for bureaucratic convenience, such as older people, people with disabilities or people with mental health problems. The worst representation of this is in oppressive language such as 'the disabled', 'the elderly' or 'the mentally ill'.
2. Workers recognise some differences, some aspects of a person's identity, and make certain assumptions and act in a particular way 'because she is a woman' or 'because he is black'.

Both of these approaches have limitations. The first, as been said, denies the personhood of the service user – and even that catch-all term is problematic. Harking back to the discussion of terminology in Chapter 3, one woman in a group discussion in a mental health hostel about users' rights stated that she did not want to be seen as someone who 'used' other people – she wanted to be called a patient. The categories acknowledge only one aspect of a person's identity and experience, and at any one time this might not be the most important aspect for them, or the one that is contributing to their needs. Using such categories might mean that the worker focuses only on this aspect of the situation.

Increasingly awareness of anti-oppressive and anti-discriminatory practice (Thompson, 1993; Dominelli, 2002b; Clifford and Burke, 2009; Bhatti-Sinclair, 2011) alerts social work practitioners to recognise other aspects of a person's experience. Most frequently this involves recognising that being a woman and/or being black significantly affects people's life experience and the way that they have been treated by health and social care services. However this sometimes happens in simplistic ways and leads to unhelpful stereotyping or unjust practices. Ahmad and Atkins (1996), for example, highlight that social workers, in recognising cultural differences, make assumptions that Asian communities look after their own and therefore packages of care are not necessary. This not only denies individuals and families services, which is unjust, it also assumes that all Asian people are the same. While it is important to respect cultural diversity it is also important to recognise the complexity of black perspectives which, according to Prevatt Goldstein (2002), consist of different interlocking experiences of each individual and have multiple expressions.

In the case of women, assumptions about women's caring capacities have locked them into caring roles, or denied them services. Just as importantly, focusing solely on women has meant that the needs of men, and the contributions that they can make to caring, have been ignored (Orme, 2001a). There are many aspects of a person's experience that should be acknowledged in assessing his/her needs and developing a package of care or working towards a personalised budget; for example his/her class, sexual orientation and/or religion. It is not appropriate to try and deny that these will make a difference to their needs – that difference includes different strengths as well as different experiences of oppression and disadvantage.

Good practice informed by social work values demands that we try to understand the diversity of service users' experience without creating a hierarchy of disadvantage. To do this it is necessary to recognise what is significant and different about these experiences, but also what is common. Most importantly, we should allow the person to express how he/she experiences the situation and what he/she wants changed. In many ways this constitutes what is known as empathy in social work – understanding the person in his/her situation.

However empathy has been criticised for being associated with professional distance and the interpretative methods of a psycho-dynamic approach. An alternative way is to think of working at borderlands (Orme, 2001a) between the person and the world as he/she experiences and interprets it. This requires that we communicate with the individual effectively, but also that we understand the discriminatory and oppressive practices and processes that he/she may be experiencing.

The notion of 'just' practice (Orme, 2002b) is associated with a person-centred approach because it avoids assumptions that a person has to be cared for, in the sense of being disempowered and/or pitied, because he/she has a set of needs. Care can be oppressive if it is assumed that people with needs are not able to think and act on their own behalf. 'Just' practice does not make any assumptions about whose needs are greater, or who is more deserving. It argues that all those who come to the attention of social services have the rights to express their needs; to have these dealt with in a fair and appropriate manner and to have effective access to resources.

Conclusion

This chapter has focused on social work with adults, concentrating on policy developments in community care including care management, person-centred planning and personalisation. It examines how social work within these policy initiatives involves many of the skills and interventions outlined in earlier chapters. It argues that social workers drawing on the value base for practice have to work with the principles of 'just' practice when responding to the needs of service users and those who provide care.

Practice focus

Mrs Short is an 89-year-old woman living in her own home in a middle-class district of a northern town. She has been widowed for over 20 years and has two sons. One lives in a nearby town and the other lives some distance away. She is fiercely independent and house-proud but has recently had an operation for a thrombosis in her arm. Just prior to being hospitalised she called out her GP because she experienced chest pains. During the visit he noticed that Mrs Short was having problems with her short-term memory, was becoming confused and the house was not as clean and organised at it usually was.

At the point of her discharge from hospital, Mrs Short was assessed for both her immediate needs and her longer-term needs. The social worker in the area team with responsibility for older people in the area was contacted by the hospital and informed of the imminent discharge. When contacting the GP's surgery the practice nurse, who was aware of the GP's concerns, conveyed these to the social worker and informed her that the GP was making a referral to the psychogeriatrician. The practice nurse also suggested that a physiotherapy assessment might be useful. She agreed to action this from the surgery.

The area had a computerised single assessment document. The social worker input the information she received into the system. This alerted her to the possible need for a home care assessment. She visited Mrs Short knowing what potential health problems she was experiencing and aware that she could get expert information about these and possible responses.

Throughout the interview Mrs Short was adamant that she did not want to leave her own home. She had been unhappy in hospital, and said she could manage with the help of relatives and neighbours. However, she did agree to a visit from the home care organiser, but expressed concern both about the cost of any services and about having no choice about who came into her home. The social worker was able to discuss personal budgets but was not totally convinced Mrs Short understood.

Once an assessment had been completed, a meeting was held at the hospital, which included health workers and Mrs Short and her son. Mrs Short was given a 'user friendly' version of the computerised assessment, but the social worker also ensured that Mrs Short understood what it was recommending.

The conclusions had been that Mrs Short was suffering early stages of vascular dementia and that she had circulatory problems which meant there was the possibility of further thrombosis. It was agreed that she would be able to stay in her own home. She would need some medical care but consideration was given to allocating her a personal budget that her son could help her administer to arrange her own care.

Point for reflection

Read the case of Mrs Short and using the principles that have been discussed in this chapter consider the approaches that could be used in this situation.

Write down how each of the principles is applied and what were the implications for Mrs Short.

What would be the advantages/disadvantages of each of these arrangements?

How do the principles of 'just' practice inform and/or influence your response to Mrs Short?

Putting it into practice

Identify a case in your practice of an adult who requires care.

1 Identify all the services and resources that the person needs to enable them to continue to live in the community, and to continue living with their quality of life.
2 Now think about what resources are available to help meet these needs. You might want to list these according to the sources e.g.:
   • the individual;
   • family;
   • friends, neighbours and other individuals in the community;
   • voluntary, independent agencies;
   • statutory services e.g. health and social services.
3 List the resources against the person's needs. Is there a mismatch? What needs are not met? Why not? Are these practical or emotional (for example, is the person lonely?) How can they be met?
4 How have different approaches, care planning, direct payments, personalisation, influenced the way that this case was handled in the agency?

Messages from research

Postle, K. (2001) 'The social work side is disappearing. I guess it started with us being called care managers', *Practice*, vol. 13, 1 pp.13–26; and Postle, K. (2002) 'Working "between the idea and the reality": ambiguities and tensions in care managers' work', *British Journal of Social Work*, vol. 32(3), pp. 335–51. Based on the author's research for her PhD these two articles give an excellent sense of the impact on social work practice of the changes brought about by care management. She argues for re-emphasising the importance of the core nature of the social work relationship.

Further resources

Carr, S. (2010) *Personalisation: a rough guide (revised edition)* Scie Report no. 20 London, Scie http://www.scie.org.uk/publications/reports/report20.pdf.
This report 'does what it says on the tin' and provides an excellent introduction to the principles of personalisation. It also gives numerous links to other relevant documents.

Gorman, H. and Postle, K. (2003) *Transforming Community Care: a distorted vision?* Birmingham: Venture Press.
A useful discussion of how practitioners have experienced care management, based on research.

Ethics and Social Welfare Journal vol. 4(2) and vol. 5(2) these two special issues on 'Care Ethics: New Theories and Applications' explore meanings of care with specific articles on, among other topics, personalisation.

Scie's e-learning resource on inter-professional and inter-agency working http://www.scie.org.uk/publications/elearning/ipiac/index.asp provides resources to explore the nature of inter-professional and inter-agency collaboration and in improving collaborative practice.

Scie's resource to assist working with carers http://www.scie.org.uk/adults/carers.asp. It includes, among other things, videos of people discussing supporting carers from a variety of perspectives.

Working with groups

CHAPTER OVERVIEW
- Theories of groupwork as a different method of intervention
- Stages of groupwork intervention
- Types and purposes of groups

Introduction

It is sometimes assumed that groupwork is any method of intervention with more than two people, but it is more than this. Theories of groupwork, drawing on social psychology, demonstrate that bringing people together in groups precipitates particular processes. Handled carefully, these processes can be powerful forces for positive change. As Trevithick (2005b) argues, the knowledge base of groupwork in social work includes three important areas: *theoretical knowledge, factual knowledge* and *practice knowledge*. The skill of good groupwork is being able to understand how these relate to each other and interweave.

This chapter will discuss some theories of groupwork and how these have influenced social work practice with groups over time.

What is different about groupwork?

One definition of a group is that it is a collection of people who spend some time together, who see themselves as members and who are identified by outsiders as members of a group (Preston-Shoot, 2007). However, group membership extends beyond the time that the members spend together: it involves a commitment and loyalty which arises out of the individual's interaction with group members and the group leader(s)/group facilitator. Also, with the introduction of social networking such as internet 'chat rooms', Facebook and similar facilities, people might consider themselves to be members of a group that is made up of people they have never physically met.

It is an interesting exercise to list the number of groups of which you are, or have been, a member. Such an exercise helps to clarify what we think we mean by a group, but also illustrates the number of different groups any one person belongs to. Both of these points are important for some of the basic theories of groupwork. For example, when we join a new work team we might not immediately feel part of the group, indeed we might feel quite excluded. What is it that eventually makes us feel that we are a member, that we have 'arrived', and why is it that some people never feel accepted – they experience exclusion? Being part of many groups causes conflicts of loyalties and confusions about behaviour. When we join a new work team we discover that tasks are done differently: systems might be better, or worse. Part of being accepted involves negotiating that fine line between holding on to the positives of our past experiences and working practices while accepting that there are things to be learned in the new situation.

These reflections help us to begin to understand the complexity of group dynamics, and give some indication of why we need to consider the literature and gain experience before undertaking groupwork. Leadership in groups involves a set of skills that may only be learned by doing. The best way to do this is to act as co-worker with an experienced groupworker, or to be a participant observer. There is a growing body of literature, including some skills manuals that involve groupwork exercises (see, for example, Doel and Sawdon, 1999), to help students of groupwork.

Groups and change

At the core of groupwork theory is the assertion that groups have the capacity to bring about change. Processes of social influence that occur in groups mean that groups bring about more lasting change than individual work (Smith, 1980). Groups provide influence by giving feedback and by providing access to coping skills. These processes are similar to Trotter's (2006) principles of prosocial modelling discussed in Chapter 9, and may be thought of as a form of behaviour modification. Smith (1980) argues that, because the range of participants in a group includes those who have similar experiences, difficulties or goals, this increases the repertoire of alternative behaviours available to the individual. Three types of social influence are significant for groupwork:

- *Compliance* occurs when a group member behaves in a way that s/he thinks is acceptable to, or desired by the group. Such change might be relatively minor and short-lived. It can also occur in individual interviews, especially as compliance occurs when one person is seen to have more control over another. In groups, individuals are often initially compliant to the leader's wishes.
- *Identification* occurs when one person is attractive to another, and the second adopts the behaviour and attitudes of the first in order to sustain a positive relationship. In that groups involve a number of participants, they provide more opportunities for identification to occur.
- *Internalisation* is seen as the most important element in group learning, and occurs when a group member makes changes because he or she observes the behaviour of someone who is attractive to him or her, and the behaviour works for him or her in his/her own situation. Again groups provide a number of opportunities to observe and test out different coping strategies.

It is useful to think about how these processes might work with different groups. For example there are risks involved in working with offenders. In the process of *identification*, if the attractive person displays anti-social or criminal behaviour there is a risk of 'contagion'. In self-help groups, these processes are very helpful in making available a range of coping mechanisms demonstrated by those in similar situations (Munn-Giddings and McVicar, 2007).

Disclosure and feedback

The process of modelling is not the only process that is enhanced by participation in a group. In all interactions we reveal something of ourselves, and as we get to know people we reveal more of ourselves. This process of disclosure happens in individual interactions, but obviously is multiplied in groups where we reveal different aspects of ourselves to different people, and in different circumstances. When we disclose aspects of ourselves, we receive feedback from others. Sometimes that is direct feedback: people tell us they agree or disagree, or indirectly by their behaviour and attitudes we discern that they do or do not like what we say or do.

Disclosure

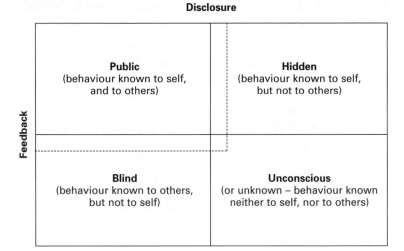

Figure 12.1 Johari window

When we receive feedback from individuals we can ignore it or perceive it as a difficulty (or a benefit) in our relationship with that individual. In groups, feedback that is received from more than one source is more difficult to ignore. Also individual group participants are more likely to give feedback in the knowledge that their views or perceptions will be supported by other group members.

The Johari window (Figure 12.1), devised by Joseph Luft and Harry Blumberg (Golembiewski and Blumberg, 1970), illustrates how this interaction of feedback and disclosure contributes to an understanding of ourselves. Either through defensiveness, lack of insight or not having been in situations before, there are aspects of our behaviour that are not apparent to us. The process of feedback, handled appropriately, helps us to understand how our behaviour impacts on others, and group situations give us the opportunity to test out how much that is a particular response from one individual, or is a more general response to our own behaviour. The experience of being in a group, of disclosing parts of ourselves and receiving feedback is therefore likely to reduce the unknown or unconscious area and contribute to insight.

Smith's (1980) notion of social influence and the processes of feedback/disclosure in the Johari window both involve change. This change is brought about by challenge and confrontation. Not in the sense of open argument and disagreement, but by individuals becoming aware of aspects of their behaviour and that of others and having to deal with it. It is the potential for change that makes groups both an effective method of intervention and a source of anxiety for both participants and groupworkers. This potential is present whatever the focus or purpose of the group, because it is the interaction between a number of different participants which provides the opportunities for feedback and insight.

The model of self-directed groupwork described by Mullender and Ward (1991) sets out with the prime aim of raising awareness and assisting users to set their own agendas for change. Even though it was not a prime aim, personal change also occurred within the members of the groups. This was mostly positive in that it enabled members to be more confident and take on more public roles.

Programmes

What is of concern, however, are developments in the use of groups that proceed on the basis of one-to-one work in groups with the rest of the group acting as bystanders (Ward, 2002). Here the emphasis is on changing behaviour by using behavioural approaches, outlined in Chapter 9, to bring about conformity. In these approaches the emphasis is on the use of the group (its members and the process) not as the instrument or medium for change, but merely as the context. Ward suggests that what he calls 'real groupwork' (see Vanstone, 2004, for some discussion) was rejected because, as is described later in this chapter, groups have a life of their own and workers do not have complete control (2002, p. 154). This was not acceptable, especially to those who were running groups as programmes designed to ensure the cessation of criminal and/or anti-social behaviour. These programmes have been introduced in criminal justice services in particular largely as a result of policy decisions (Vanstone, 2004). They are thought to be a more effective use of workers' time, and help to standardise practice. Packages (of exercises to work with, for example, perpe-trators of domestic violence, or those convicted of drink-driving offences) have been accredited for use throughout criminal justice agencies as part of the 'what works' agenda, that is, they were thought to be effective and it was policy that they should be used with all offenders.

Brown (2002), in discussing the tension between processes and packages, suggests that workers welcome packages because they give them some sense of control, while group members welcome this approach because it takes away the sense of responsibility that they might have to participate. However, working unreflectively with these packages can mean that opportunities for effective intervention may be lost. More problematic is that the group might become totally disruptive, with negative effects on its members.

Ward has suggested changes in groupwork practice relate to the 'demethoding' of social work (Ward, 2009), that is a move away from traditional skills and interventions. However, a UK survey (Doel and Sawdon, 2001) found a commitment to using groupwork: a high proportion of respondents were workers in criminal justice agencies. They might therefore be involved in delivering packages or accredited groupwork programmes which might support Ward's analysis but Doel and Sawdon argue that there is evidence of immense complexity of groups and groupwork. This is supported by descriptions of groupwork approaches in a variety of contexts (see for example Cohen and Mullender, 2003).

Types and purposes of groups

Now that we have been critical of a programmatic approach to groupwork, it is necessary to explore what Ward (2002) means by 'real' groupwork. In the first instance, this involves looking at different kinds of groups, and their purposes. It helps to understand that group aims usually prescribe the type and methods to use. Different purposes of groups are those broadly categorised as remedial, reciprocal and social goals models (Papell and Rothman, 1966). Other categories distinguish between social or recreational groups, group psychotherapy, group counselling, educational groups, social treatment groups (for example, sex offender groups), discussion groups, self-help groups, social action groups (for example, welfare rights), and self-directed groups (for example, campaigning or other objectives decided by the members).

The reason why groups fail to 'get going' might be related to how they are formed, composed and led, but also a failure to be clear about purposes. During its lifetime a group may change its purposes, for instance from discussion to campaigning. Unless it is openly stated at the outset what the purposes are, groups can 'lose their way' and become very puzzling for their members. One group, supposedly a recreational one for single-parent mothers, had a hidden agenda aimed at getting the women to improve their parenting skills, so it was doomed from the start. Whitaker (1975) gives four conditions for successful groupwork:

- Success is more likely if other people in the agency support the group purpose and procedures. Sabotage is also less likely.
- A group is more likely to be effective if a consensus can be established within the group about aims and methods.
- Structural factors such as size, duration, composition, constancy of membership and ratio of staff to members influence effectiveness.
- A group that has lost its purpose should be reconstituted with a different mandate or terminated.

This underlines the need for commitment to groupwork by the individual worker and the agency. The only reason for using groupwork, as opposed to any other practice method, is that it is the best way of helping the people concerned, not because the workers want to try it or because it is an economical way of offering a service.

Groups have their disadvantages, not least that some individuals are frightened of them. This fear is linked to a sense of ambivalence; of wanting to belong to the group but being afraid that the group might require giving up autonomy: asking members to do or think something with which they do not agree. On the other hand, groups can be a source of power for individuals pressing for social change. They can provide mutual support, opportunities for exchange of information and motivate hope. The use of groups in criminal justice services also demonstrates how groups can be used for education (for example alcohol awareness and impaired drivers courses), or confronting unacceptable behaviour (for example anger management and offending behaviour groups). Groups offer the opportunity to learn and test interpersonal and other social skills; they offer a sense of belonging and 'being in the same boat' which is reassuring. There is scope to use the leader or other members as role models and to get feedback about coping attempts. Perhaps, most significantly, there is a chance to help as well as be helped.

Mullender and Ward (1991) describe what they call empowering groupwork. In this they see social justice as paramount in ensuring that:

- all people have skills, understanding and ability;
- people have rights to be heard, to participate, to choose, to define problems and action;

- people's problems are complex and social oppression is a contributory factor;
- people acting collectively are powerful: methods of work must be non-elitist and non-oppressive.

This empowering approach can be used in groups facilitated by workers but also has implications for the types of group, e.g. user-led groups.

Planning the group

Once the type and broad aims of the group have been decided on, a major task is planning and preparation. Questions to be answered in the planning process include:

- *Who?* The composition of a group may already be determined, such as those in hospital wards, residential and day centres and neighbourhoods. However, even when the qualification for the group membership is obvious, attention has to be paid to diversity and balance. These have to reflect the needs of the members and the purpose of the group. Race and gender are obvious categories (Cohen and Mullender, 2003) but other differences such as age and commonality of need can also be important.
- *How many?* The question of group size depends on the aims of the group, but usually there needs to be more than three and less than fourteen people, what Brown (1992) suggests is 'large enough for stimulation, small enough for participation and recognition'.
- *How long?* Open-ended or time limited? Open or closed membership? All such decisions relate to the aims and purpose of the particular group. Open groups are those that can be joined at any time. Closed groups have a selected membership at the outset, are time-limited and do not allow people to join during the lifetime of the group. In settings such as hospitals or prisons there is often little choice, as the movement of patients, prisoners and staff on shift systems dictates membership. The length of each session needs to be considered too, for instance work with children, older people and those who are frail requires short sessions with rest breaks.
- *Which methods?* The methods must suit the members, skills of the leader(s) and the stated aims. It may be that it is only when

the group has met that final decisions can be taken. Methods may include a variety of games, discussions, activities, experiential exercises and entertainments, depending on resources available. Methods might also be dictated by agency policy, or by the specification of the court, as in the case of a violent offender who receives a community supervision sentence that involves attending an anger-management group.

- *What resources?* There are a number of practical issues to be addressed such as: Is there a meeting place? Is transport available if necessary? Will refreshments be provided? What equipment is needed, and so on? For groups with special needs appropriate accommodation and support systems will be required. For example, some people with disabilities are accompanied by care assistants who will assist with practical tasks; older people with hearing difficulties may need someone to sit with them to ensure they hear all that is going on. Resources have to be mediated with the agency. This may include providing a breakdown of costs in terms of time spent, staffing by one leader or two, if an outside consultant is to be used, what recording systems will be used and if workers in the whole team can make referrals, for instance from their current workloads.

Groupworkers can draw on a variety of theories to help them in their approach. Most groupworkers draw on theories of social psychology to help make their decisions about size, composition, leadership, power and influence. Social psychology also informs understandings of stages of group development.

Stages of group development and the worker's tasks

Groups evolve through stages during which the behaviour of the members, the leader's interventions and the accomplishment of tasks or activities can be affected. Following individual 'screening' (for group members and workers) a groupworker has to follow the energy of the group through trust, challenge, openness, interdependence and finally independence. At different stages, the worker has to be central, pivotal, peripheral and central once again. Accordingly, the worker is in tune with the stages of group development known as forming, storming, norming, performing and adjourning (Tuckman and Jensen, 1977).

Other groupwork theorists name these stages differently, but all agree the phenomena to be observed at each: Yalom (1970) describes orientation, conflict then cohesiveness; Schutz (1966) outlines cycles when the group is concerned with inclusion, control and affection, while Whitaker (1985) talks about formative, established and termination phases.

Forming

In the forming stages, members move quickly from orientation and exploration, in which there is parallel communication aimed at the worker, to more communications with each other. The group and the worker are tested to see if trust can be established. The tasks for the practitioner are to help people to get involved, to link people and their common concerns, and to encourage the development of a group bond. When people join a group they want to know if the sacrifice of their individual wants will be compensated by the benefits of joining the group. The worker takes any opportunity to point out how members, sharing similar interests and problems, are in a position to understand and thereby help one another. To summarise some of the skills and tasks of the leader in the early meetings:

- Give a short presentation of yourself.
- Ask members to do the same.
- Review information given to members prior to joining.
- Amend any aims and agreements.
- Acknowledge initial uncertainties.
- Get each person to say what he or she hopes to get out of the group.
- Summarise issues as presented.
- Establish norms for listening and accepting.
- Facilitate interaction: 'Does anybody else feel the same?'.
- Play the absent member role, putting into words what people may want to say but are not yet ready to risk.
- Show concern for each individual.
- Balance answering questions with 'Does anyone else know the answer to that?'

(Northen, 1969; Heap, 1985)

Storming

During the storming stage, subgroups and pairings may have formed (later, these relationships extend to include the whole group). It is a stage characterised by the replacement of 'Do I belong?' with 'Do I have any influence?' Struggles for power and control underlie communications, and there is a tendency for members to polarise around certain issues. Further exploring and testing takes place: the group is quite fragile and may not continue if the leadership does not provide enough security while individuals question if they are going to get what they came for. This stage can be draining. Some skills and tasks are:

• Keep calm in the face of member–member, member–leader conflicts.
• Do not retaliate when your authority is challenged; it may stem from ambivalence about membership or a transference reaction.
• Model acceptance and openly recognise that people are different.
• Do not pick out isolated or difficult members for attention.
• Try to pace and time when to facilitate and when to be quiet.
• Begin to release responsibilities to the membership.

Norming

The norming stage indicates that group cohesion is established; members may express intimate and personal opinions to each other. People start to look for 'affection', that is, signs that the wider group accepts them. Cooperation, sharing information and decision making by consensus promote synergistic (the extra power of combined action) outcomes. People identify with the group and its future: a 'we' feeling develops, a growing *esprit de corps*. A norm of high attendance, ritual ownership of seats and some exclusivity is likely to make it difficult for new members to join. A lack of conformity to group norms can lead to scapegoating or group pressure to conform. New leadership from within the group may result in altering basic group norms. For the worker, the tasks are to:

• Let people help each other by stepping out of a directing role into a listening, following one.
• Be pivotal when observing and commenting on what seems to be happening, asking the group what their perceptions are as well as offering ideas of your own.
• Be more aware of process as well as content. It helps to ask oneself (and perhaps the group), 'What is going on here? What is this issue really all about?' in order to help people to express feelings and challenge comments.

Performing

When performing occurs, this means that the group has developed a culture of acting together to solve problems: it is no longer the leader's group; rather the workers become peripheral as the members perceive that 'this is our group'. Individual and group goals are tackled, meaning that members model coping mechanisms and values for each other. A high-status or charismatic member may further enhance a group's willingness to let individuals 'try on' different roles, thus preparing for eventual differentiation and independence from the group. In one group a member, who could be relied on as 'competent and responsible', acted as a facilitator for the rest and bravely pointed out that sometimes he did not feel confident and would prefer sometimes to take a break from feeling responsible. The worker:

• observes how the group handle each other and the tasks;
• gives ideas when these are sought;
• shows interest and expresses praise and appreciation of efforts;
• continues to model in relation to confidence, attitudes and problem solving.

Adjourning

The adjourning or ending stage usually follows the achievement of the task, and requires disengagement from relationships. All groups have to end some time, otherwise they risk stagnation or low productivity. Imposed time limits can prevent the worker from hanging on to a group merely because he/she feels guilty or uncertain about 'letting go'. There will be a sense of loss and maybe rejection and attempts to continue the group, despite agreed parameters, but, with good leadership, ultimately, acceptance and a sense of achievement. The worker, more active again, can do these things:

• set goals for the time left in partnership with the group;
• review experiences, emphasising gains as well as feelings of loss;
• reinforce interests outside the group;
• help the group to return to the planning stage if they want to continue but with some other purpose;
• evaluate the sessions and ask for feedback.

Handling difficulties in groups

Describing group development through the above phases might suggest that all is straightforward and predictable when, in reality, stages only represent tendencies from which any group can veer. In addition, it is interesting to note that each time a group meets it goes through some version of these stages, in that each meeting brings people together, and requires them to negotiate the tasks and then prepare to end.

Understanding these processes has to be accompanied by recognition of what Heap (1985) calls 'latent' communication in groups. Often, there are recurring themes: for instance when a group seems preoccupied with a particular, apparently irrelevant topic. This might mistakenly be ignored instead of associated with something people cannot talk about directly. This is referred to as a common group tension or focal conflict. Recognising the deeper meaning of content and managing the processes around focal conflicts takes sensitivity and advanced skills.

Beyond symbolic communication difficulties, workers fantasise about the possibility that a group will simply take no notice of the leader or that strong emotions will result in chaos and damaged individuals. Even experienced workers are anxious when a group member is isolated, scapegoated, speaks too much or too little. Generally, many of these difficulties can be put back to the group for their resolution; otherwise individual counselling might help, or it may be that the behaviour is needed by the group for some reason and should be explored (see Doel and Sawdon, 1999, for discussion of techniques).

Roles in groups

The *scapegoat* phenomenon is when a person is ostracised by the group and held responsible for what is going wrong in the group. The leader should avoid siding with or against the scapegoat, and ask the group to reflect on what is happening. If the scapegoat does not need protection or mediation, the leader can attempt to reduce guilt, fear or whatever feelings the group are suppressing and projecting on to one member by talking about such feelings in a general way. For example, in student groups one person may be aggressive and outspoken; the rest hide their feelings so as not to be different or unpopular. It is possible to point out that what the outspoken student is saying is felt by a lot of people even though they may not admit it. Reflection on how social workers may fear conflict and how dealing with it is an issue every day in practice can help free the group from unhelpful patterns.

The *monopoliser* is when someone dominates in the group. If it is not dealt with this behaviour can cause other members to absent themselves or explode! The problem with allowing someone to dominate a group is that this stops others with useful things to say from contributing. Intervention has to take place early on to prevent group structure hardening, and while the leader still has patience. For example, in a group of carers one man went on at length about his experience. As this was the first meeting he might have overwhelmed other participants with his knowledge and so, having thanked him for prompting the group to explore a range of ideas, the worker indicated clearly that she would like to hear everyone's point of view.

Silent members can cause resentment because some groups resent it if a person stays silent believing that the person is quietly judging them or not sharing. However, there may be complex other reasons for silence. Teasing silent members or saying 'We haven't heard from you, Mrs Brown,' is not helpful. A more positive intervention is something along the lines of, 'I remember you said something about this once, Mrs Brown. Could you remind us about your suggestion as I think it would help?' Conveying an interest in hearing from people and modelling respect can also be done non-verbally with a touch, gesture or eye contact – swivelling one's eyes around a student group will usually catch a reticent person who might speak if encouraged with a nod.

Obviously, there cannot be prescriptions for handling all the problems that arise. It is important to use supervision and 'wash-up' sessions (that is, sessions held immediately after the group to reflect on what has gone on) to identify what has worked, and what has not.

Co-leadership

Problems are also easier to handle if there is co-leadership of the group. Arguments for co-leading or co-facilitating include: handling large groups; continuity when one leader is absent; managing when members get out of control or express strong emotions; and when work is to be done in subgroups (Preston-Shoot, 2007). Planning, selecting and presenting a co-leader to the group should include consideration of gender and race combinations. Groupwork is demanding, and few of us are able to concentrate all the time. Co-working allows the responsibility for taking the initiative to be shared. On these occasions the other person can observe and reflect on the group processes as they occur. This dynamic can provide valuable feedback to the group itself while it is in process, and to the co-worker in the post-group discussions or 'wash-up'. There could be disadvantages when the co-workers hold widely differing views on goals and styles and when the sole worker already has the resources required. These can be overcome by careful selection of co-workers, and can be dealt with in supervision.

Practice focus

A criminal justice team set up a group for men who had been sentenced for offences of domestic violence. A team of workers operated in pairs (one male and one female worker) to offer different modules of a programme that had been approved by the Home Office. The programme consisted of six modules, each of five weeks' duration. Men referred to the group by the courts were expected to attend all the sessions as part of their supervision order. Failure to attend the group could lead to a man being taken back to the court and sentenced for the original offence, which might entail a custodial sentence. Each of the modules had a predefined set of tasks and exercises relating to particular themes. The format also required that the men acknowledged their violence, and the group opened each week with the members having to indicate if they had had violent feelings. Group leaders were expected to challenge any behaviour and attitudes that might demean or threaten women.

Part way through the second module of the programme a particular session was extremely difficult for the group leaders to manage. The men were initially silent and refusing to participate in the exercises arranged by the group leaders. When challenged by the leaders for non-compliance the men became vociferous and argumentative. They said that they felt the group leaders were abusing their power, and that this was ironic when the men themselves were being asked to reflect on their own use of power and control. They also complained that they were being asked to reveal in public (in front of other members of the group) things that they considered personal and confidential.

The group leaders had to abandon the exercises planned for that evening and to try to resolve some of the strong feelings. It became apparent that not all the men shared the views expressed but that some particularly strong members dominated and others felt that they had to comply.

In supervision after this session the group leaders, who were both qualified social workers, were able to acknowledge that in running this 'course' they had ignored the fact that they were in fact running a 'group'. Despite being aware of the theory and practice of group processes they had been deterred from thinking about groupwork theory because it was associated with 'therapy' and they were not running a therapeutic group. However, the fact that the same group of men were meeting together on a regular basis for a particular purpose meant group processes had been operating but had not been considered by the group leaders. Classic roles had been undertaken by the men. By not observing these or the processes of influence, the group leaders had not anticipated how the dynamics of the group had developed and were getting in the way of the purpose of the group.

Recording

In relation to recording, some groupworkers keep a register showing standard information such as date, session number, members and leaders present/absent, plan for the session, what happened (that is, content and process), and an evaluation of what went well and what did not (Brown, 1992). Others use visual means: a seating plan is drawn with a series of circles representing each member. In a more complex recording method, the circles are divided into three portions indicating the beginning, middle and end of the session, noting atmosphere, influence, participation, tasks and decision making at each time stage in the 'interaction chronogram'. Other methods include a pro forma where leaders write short notes about each participant at the end of the session. These methods can reflect the group process and are useful when the worker and co-worker review the session, prepare for the next and make appropriate interventions related to specific group members.

However, where groups involve members who are on the case-loads of other workers, systems have to be agreed for giving feedback to colleagues, which do not breach any confidentiality agreements the group may have agreed. Also, there should be agreement in advance what arrangements there will be for contacting individuals who have indicated specific problems that have not been, or cannot be, dealt with in the group.

Finally, groups that operate to enable members to fulfil the requirements of court orders have to develop agreed recording methods that both respect the members of the group, and fulfil the requirements of the court.

Conclusion

This chapter has set out the theory that informs the practice of running groups. This has implications for the purpose, organisation, membership, and leadership of groups. It has been suggested that whatever the focus of a particular group, there are certain dynamics that occur which should be incorporated into the work with the group. To do this means that the group itself becomes an important and effective medium for bringing about change. If such dynamics are ignored this does not just constitute lost opportunties, it means that sometimes the intended outcomes of the work will not be achieved. It will be counter-productive.

Point for reflection

We are all members of different groups at different times in our lives. We can therefore learn about groups from observing and reflecting on our own experiences.

1 List some of the groups that you have been a member of (see if you can think of about six different groups). Some might be formal ones such as work teams or sports groups; others might be informal such as friendship groups. Then there are 'natural' groups such as families.

2 Now, using what you have read in this chapter try to identify what was significant about each of these groups. Was it the membership? The purpose? How do you think this group influenced you? Why do you think this happened?

Putting it into practice

In your practice prepare for a meeting or group session that you are going to participate in. Work out how you will make observations about the processes that the meeting or group goes through. While you are in the group or the meeting identify what roles people take on and how that facilitates or blocks the processes. Don't forget to observe your own role. You might want to discuss the possibility of sharing your observations – having an observer can influence the group dynamics, even if the members do not know they are being observed.

Messages from research

Munn-Giddings, C. and McVicar, A. (2006) 'Self-help groups as mutual support: What do carers value?', *Health and Social Care in the Community*, 15(1), 26–34 This research used semi-structure interviews to explore the experiences of carers in groups. It concludes that self-help/mutual aid groups, based on reciprocal peer support, offer a valuable type of resource in the community that is not replicable in professional–client relations.

Further resources

Cohen, M. and Mullender, A. (eds) (2003) *Gender and Groupwork*. London: Routledge.
This text describes groupwork with women in a number of different contexts.

Doel, M. and Sawdon, C. (1999) *The Essential Groupwork: teaching and learning creative groupwork*. London: Jessica Kingsley.
A very useful text that incorporates exercises as well as explaining the theory of groupwork.

Vanstone, M.T. (2003) 'A History of the Use of Groups in Probation Work: Part One – from "Clubbing the Unclubbables" to "Therapeutic Intervention"', *Howard Journal*, 42(1), pp. 69–86.
This first of two articles traces the development of groupwork in probation work as an important part of the theory and practice of supervising probationers in the community. As such, it gives a useful summary of the use of groupwork in social work.

Vanstone, M. (2004) 'A History of the Use of Groups in Probation Work: Part Two – From Negotiated Treatment to Evidence Based Practice in an Accountable Service', *The Howard Journal of Criminal Justice*, 43(2), pp. 180–222.
This second article argues for the relevance of work with groups, and how such work encouraged a more collaborative approach focused more specifically on the offence. It explores the changing

use of groupwork influenced by both evidence-based practice and increased governance both of probationers and of probation policy and practice.

The website of the Association of Advancement of Social Work with Groups http://www.aaswg.org/ provides useful resources and discussion about developments in groupwork.

CHAPTER 13

Working with communities

Introduction

A dwindling emphasis on working with communities in statutory work during the 1980s led to suggestions that community work is not part of social work. However, community work has always been part of wider definitions of social work which, with individual work and groupwork, involves a 'holy trinity' of approaches. Community work can be a distinct form of practice and calls upon a theoretical and knowledge base that is more sociological and less psychological than individual work and groupwork (Payne, 1995). However, this chapter argues that this knowledge base informs practice in and with communities in a variety of ways. In addition, because community approaches in social work require a change of emphasis from individual to community and collective (Ferguson and Woodward, 2009), they should be an integral part of empowering social work. The chapter starts however by discussing the contested nature of the term community.

Community

Many attempts have been made to define communities, most of which include notions of size and place. This might include a very large group; a locality which might include street, town or city boundaries; or a society which can be regional, national and international (as in the European Community).

The notion of community is, therefore, one of the most contested within sociological literature. While there are often common elements in definitions (locality, attachment, shared interests) there is little agreement on the relative significance of any of these elements (for further discussion, see Henderson and Thomas, 1981; Allen, 1991; and Orme 2001a).

Two basic distinctions highlight the complexities of defining community:

- *Community as locality*: sometimes called community of residence, where place is both synonymous with community and influences those who live in the community. The individual is expected to share things in common with others living in the same geographical area, and to feel some loyalty to that area and its inhabitants. Relationships develop (some positive, some antagonistic). The lifestyle adopted by those living in the community may be influenced by the views of others in that locality. The individual will be part of many networks of relationships whose focus is on the local area. It is these local networks of formal and informal relationships together with their capacity to mobilise individual and collective responses that constitute a sense of community.
- *Community of interest*: functional communities exist because individuals also have a number of relationships with people and institutions outside a circumscribed geographical area. Their common interest may be based on leisure or work, and these networks of relationships might extend even beyond national boundaries. For example, international associations of social workers constitute a community with a shared interest in the profession of social work. Shared interests might also arise out of a particular social disadvantage, hence the Disability Rights Movement constitutes a community of interest which has a national context but also has links with groups experiencing similar disadvantage in other countries.

Over time, these distinctions have been challenged. The mobility of individuals and families due to economic changes and the use of communication technology have meant that networks are maintained in a variety of ways. Clubs and activities for people based on their place of origin, for example Ireland, Scotland or the West Indies, allowed for a celebration of characteristics related to place in a quite different geographic location. Advances in communication using different technologies have led to enormous increases in communities of interest. This might suggest that we either abandon the notion of community, or widen the definition.

For the purposes of working with communities, a useful definition focuses on the conditions necessary for effective interventions for, and by, communities in order to bring about change or 'realise' the community. In this approach a community is:

- a unit large enough to be a political force and small enough to account for, and relate to, the individual person;
- an optimal location to develop alternative models of social (and economic) organisation;
- a point of mobilisation of people to effect social change that can be self-organised;
- a unit of people that can command sufficient resources to establish alternative institutional arrangements;
- a unit for analysis that will identify the forces and material conditions determining social relations. (provided by the Non-Violence Study Group and quoted in Thomas, 1983)

Thomas argues that it is the concept of 'neighbourhood' that has most influenced community work. He argues that, based on geographical areas, neighbourhoods may contain 'different intensities of networks that express people's support, care, trust, and responsibilities and obligations to one another' (Thomas, 1983, p. 173). This notion of 'networks' has become significant in the development of social work with communities and is now relevant to both actual (geographical) and virtual communities.

Community in social work

The relationship of social work with community work is a complex one. Historically social work had close associations with community work. Howe (1992) identifies collective action as forming part of the methods of socialist welfare work (alongside fighting for rights and entitlements and arguing that social problems are the consequences of a capitalist economy). Feminist writers, while critiquing developments in community work and social work, point out that mobilising strengths and resources in collectives arose out of the women's movement (Dominelli and McLeod, 1989).

The introduction of community care led to redefinitions of the community in social work (Smale *et al.*, 1988) and radical critiques

(Ferguson and Woodward, 2009) have led to a resurgence of interest in community development.

Community development

The most active phase of relationships between social work and community work was the 1960s. The national community development projects (CDP) were set up by the Home Office Children's Departments, and community development workers were employed who were independent of the newly created social services departments. Workers were to be active, mobilising resources within the community. The focus was on organising local communities and improving coordination between welfare agencies. The work undertaken included:

- individual welfare rights
- advocacy
- surveys
- campaigning
- community self-help projects (for example, advice centres, adventure playgrounds, women's refuges)

These tasks, often called community action, involved work with community groups and using collective approaches to resolve problems, even if the problems were being experienced primarily by individuals. Those engaged in various forms of community work were 'concerned with affecting the course of social change through the two processes of analysing social situation and forming relationships with different groups to bring about desirable change' (Calouste Gulbenkian Foundation, 1968, p. 4).

This approach to community work is described by Mayo (2002) as the process of assisting ordinary people to improve their own communities by collective action. In doing this, community workers attempted to understand situations in terms of not only who holds the power but also whose interests are served by particular policies and practices.

Focusing on the community rather than the individual was seen to be a positive move away from casework, which was why it became seen as separate from social work rather than an extension of it. However community work was not a panacea. There is a danger that a community, rather than the individual could be pathologised and experienced as the problem (Loney, 1983): for example, labelling some areas as 'sink estates'. Another danger is that community work can be employed as a palliative when the substantial resources needed to overcome major injustices were not forthcoming (Popple, 1995, p. 27). This is a particular risk if community work focuses on communities 'making do' with poor conditions rather than advocating, for example, better housing, local health and education resources.

These dangers highlight competing perspectives on, or traditions in, the role of community work. These are alternatively defined as the differences between the (political) left and right (Mayo, 2002), or the differences between top-down and bottom-up community action (Popple, 2002). An alternative distinction is:

• The liberal approach to community work, which is about promoting self-help and improving services delivery within the existing frameworks. Such an approach can be seen in political rhetoric about the 'big society' or the 'good society'. This approach has also been labelled as a professional or technicist approach.
• The radical, or transformational, approach to community work, which tries to shift the balance of social relations by empowering the powerless to question the causes of their deprivation and challenge the sources of their oppression. (Mayo, 2002, p. 165)

These distinctions, often highlighted by the different focus and locus of activity, influence the way that community work is undertaken.

The different approaches also have repercussions for those undertaking the work. Community action approaches involved emerging voluntary groups who worked with local community groups, particularly in working-class areas, to fight local causes. Definitional distinctions emerged that separated community work, which was undertaken by those paid to do it, and community action, which was undertaken by those in conflict with authority. These distinctions led to debate in the 1970s about whether community workers should become a separate profession, and whether there was scope for radical activities by those undertaking community work in statutory agencies, including social work agencies.

Community work therefore operates in a number of different ways. As well as being a form of intervention it is:

• an *attitude* that defines a more participative and egalitarian set of relations;

- associated with a *critique* of existing power and resources;
- a *principle* of service delivery, making local services relevant, accessible and accountable to their users;
- a *frame of reference* and identification of like-minded people;
- a *work site* for those professionals who do their job 'in' the community (as opposed to an office). (Thomas, 1983)

Tasks and skills

Popple (2002) argues that a generic bottom-up definition of community work is working with people using skills, information and strategies in ways that encourage them to do things for themselves. However, historically the identification of tasks and skills for community work tends to reflect the tension between liberal/radical and top-down/bottom-up approaches.

For example, early models of community organisation and intervention (Rothman, 1968) included social planning, locality development and social action. Social action was closer to social work as it was about direct work with people, particularly those identified as having, or joining together because of, mutual interests or oppressions. In systems terms, the power structure is assumed to lie outside the client system (in this case the community) and is therefore an external target of action, but the intervention is top-down.

York (1984) developed a different framework for theorising community work, or community social work, as he calls it. He focuses on the differences between *directive* and *non-directive intervention*. The distinctions reflect the primary goals of the workers and what they want to achieve rather than roles that they adopt at any one time in their work. These echo top-down/bottom-up distinctions:

- *Directive intervention*: involves the agency deciding, more or less specifically, what it thinks the clients need, what they ought to value or what they ought to do, and even, at times, how they ought to behave.
- *Non-directive intervention*: the worker does not attempt to decide for people or to lead, guide or persuade them to accept her/his specific conclusions about what is good for them, but works to get them to decide for themselves what their needs are. The worker's role is to provide favourable conditions for successful action by strengthening and stimulating incentive,

providing information, helping community members to analyse problems systematically.

A model of how different approaches would be viewed is given below, although York (1984) emphasises that this is a continuum of activity, rather than a set of opposites:

Directive intervention	*Non-directive intervention*
Task approach	Problem approach
Initiating roles	Enabling roles
Treatment	Reform

Another way of analysing community work intervention draws on understandings of systems (see Chapter 3) and involves identifying the different arenas in which community workers are involved, and in which they might use the methods discussed above. These arenas, or parts of the system, involve negotiations with different people and it is these negotiations that provide the focus for activity. For Henderson and Thomas (1981) these arenas include:

1. Transactions with local people, either as individuals or in group situations. These might be tenants, parents, health care users or residents of a particular street.
2. Transactions between the group and other systems in its environment. These other systems are difficult to predict and might involve other local residents, representatives of official bodies, such as the housing authority, or politicians.
3. Transactions about the group within the worker's own agencies. Recognising that, for example, social work services might need to change, the worker has to be advocate as well as change agent.

Drawing on group processes, Henderson and Thomas (1981) identify seven types of interventions/discussions that exemplify non-directive approaches in community work. Although the functions need to be performed in community work with local people (or neighbourhood work) they do not all have to be undertaken by the same person. While others can undertake the tasks/interventions, the community worker needs to ensure that the relevant processes occur. They include:

- galvanising
- focusing
- clarifying
- summarising

- gatekeeping
- mediating
- informing

The community worker becomes a director – and when working at the interface between local people and more formal and established organisations, the community worker also has to ensure that a number of other functions are carried out, which include broker, mediator, advocate, negotiator and bargainer. Again, different people can perform these functions but thought has to be given to what role will be played by which individuals, because balance has to be struck between the appropriate activity for the paid worker and the community members. It would be possible for workers to perform all these tasks using skills, processes and interventions that are core to social work. However, they have to be shared. The paid worker might act in some form of representative role for the group or community at, for example, town or city council meetings or inter-views with local authority officers. Or when community members take lead roles the paid worker might have a set of facilitative func-tions, which include observer/recorder, delegate or plenipotentiary.

It is important to remember that power operates in all sorts of subtle ways. While it might seem appropriate to hand power over to the community, there is a risk that individuals might dominate in communities, but might not represent the views of the majority. This is particularly important as communities are becoming increasingly diverse. Often the role of mediator within communi-ties is necessary if, for example, there are strong negative feelings expressed towards immigrant groups or to the settlement of asylum seekers. Workers need to ensure that as many people as possible feel included, and have their voices heard.

Mayo sums up the skills for community work as including:

- engagement (with individuals, groups and organisations)
- assessment (including area profiles)
- research
- groupwork
- negotiation
- communication
- counselling
- management of resources
- resourcing (for example grant applications)
- recording and report writing (for a wide range of audiences)
- monitoring and evaluation. (Mayo, 2002, p. 16)

While community work might not necessarily be carried out by those employed in statutory social work agencies, workers undertaking community work draw on skills that are core to the social work profession. This is the complex relationship between social work and community work.

One of the main distinctions between the two has been said to be where the work actually takes place, that is, in a community rather than in a social work agency. However this takes us back to the discussion of what is meant by 'community'.

Community care

The language of *community* care suggests social workers should engage with communities. In a review of the role and tasks of social work, the Barclay Committee (1982) made a distinction between community work and social work. The committee claimed that community work embraced both direct work with community groups and work at the inter-organisational and planning level by influencing policies. They concluded that, 'This work can be an element of social work, but it does not include the whole of social work, nor does social work embrace the whole of community work' (Barclay, 1982, p. xiii).

However, later policy agendas of social inclusion suggest that even if social workers are working with individuals and families they need to be alert to both the pressures and the opportunities that work with communities offers. Policy developments around personalisation, as we saw in Chapter 11, suggest that work has to be done with communities to ensure service user access to resources. Therefore it could be argued that even if social workers do not 'do' community work, they have to work with community workers to ensure that service users are not excluded from communities. Community work has been, by definition, particularly concerned with the needs of those who have been disadvantaged or oppressed, whether through poverty, or through discrimination on the basis of race, class, gender, sexuality, age or disability (Mayo, 1994). In acknowledging and developing some of the skills of community work, social workers might be more effective in fighting oppression.

However, separating discussion of community care from community work serves to highlight that the policies of community care do not necessarily depend upon understandings of community work. The original philosophy of community care, focusing on individuals with need and meeting these needs with individualised packages of care, paid little heed to any of the various definitions that recognise the radical potential of communities. Community care policies reflect a limited, liberal, top-down approach to communities. They require activities that ensure not only that needs of people in the community are understood but also that individuals, groups and organisations within communities are prepared, and able, to provide caring services and facilities (Orme and Glastonbury, 1993). There were serious question raised about whether 'community care' as reflected in the policies required care *in* the community, or care by the community (Orme, 2001a).

Similar questions can be asked about personalisation where policies assert that those who require community care services have to be treated as full and active members of communities capable of both providing and receiving services. However, critiques of personalisation suggest that the policies have not actively acknowledged the different definitions of communities and the diversity within communities discussed above.

However discussions within community care did lead to interesting work around community social work.

Community social work

The Barclay Committee gave a conservative definition of community social work (as opposed to community work) as:

> formal social work which, starting from the problems affecting an individual or group and the responsibilities and resources of social services departments and voluntary organisations, seeks to tap into, support, enable and underpin the local networks of formal and informal relationships which constitute our basic definition of community, and also the strengths of a client's communities of interest. (Barclay, 1982, p. xvii)

An appendix to the main report (Appendix A) described a 'patch' approach that would enable workers to work with local resources to provide 'neighbourhood clusters' of formal and informal care. This would involve personal social services in:

• working in close collaboration with informal caring networks;
• finding ways of developing partnerships between informal carers (including self-help groups), statutory services and voluntary agencies;

- ensuring ready access of caring networks to statutory and voluntary services;
- offering those who give and receive services opportunities to share decisions which affect their lives. (Barclay, 1982, para. 13.13)

Such activities could be seen to be a pre-cursor to the personalisation agenda but the approach was seen to be instrumental – the emphasis is not on communities as sites of action but as sources of care provision. The move towards a mixed economy of welfare in later community care legislation meant that communities were seen as replacements for state providers, not sources of innovation and challenge.

Smale *et al.* (1988) offer a different scenario. They see Barclay and Appendix A as reflecting the development of community social work as localisation. They suggest a shift of focus to the relationships between people, and the patterns of these relationships. Social workers should manage change through innovation in practice. Their view of community social work is that it involves a process of working out aims and objectives through a review of needs and resources with a wide range of people. This is dependent, not on where the work happens, but how. It is the *processes* the workers engage in and the *relationships* they make and how these are maintained and changed that is important (Smale *et al.*, 1988, p. 23).

In focusing on processes and relationships, Smale *et al.* do not prescribe specific sets of skills, or methods that could or should be used in 'doing' community social work. The whole emphasis of the 'approach' is that methods, skills and actions will evolve from the focus of the team of social workers identifying both what resources they have available within themselves and the 'community' and what is required. However, they do list areas where more emphasis might be required:

- working across agency boundaries
- working on the margins of complex systems
- working in teams of peers and others
- working in ways open to public accountability
- working with devolved responsibilities and budgets
- working in networks of partnership
- working to understand sequences of behaviour that perpetuate problems and intervening to change these patterns. (Smale *et al.*, 1988)

Community development revisited

Recent debates in social work about communities have returned to the more radical approaches to working with communities associated with community development. Although the funded Community Development Projects (CDP) were abandoned in the 1970s, the principles have continued, especially in Scotland. For example the Scottish Community Development Centre (SCDC) sees community development as an approach that strengthens local democracy and the capacity and voice of communities to participate actively in determining the processes and outcomes of social and economic change (Barr, Drysdale *et al.*, 1998). The aim is to try to achieve change through rational discourse, fostering collective values and moral persuasion (Popple, 1995, p. 41). These principles have been translated into radical approaches to community work, where the aim is to change the balance and structure of social relations informed by the causes of oppression, rather than merely change the mode of service delivery. Importantly, community development is not exclusive to social work, but nor is social work excluded from it.

Community development and social work

Ife (2002) writing about community development and social work describes it as the process of establishing or re-establishing structures of human community within which new ways of relating, organising social life and meeting human needs become possible. This might suggest the end of social work as we know it, but more positively it has stimulated changes related to user participation and empowerment that emphasise a different relationship between those in need of services and agencies that exist to meet those needs. In Scotland, the *Changing Lives* report (Scottish Executive, 2006a) calls for a 'new approach', which positions social work services at the heart of communities (p. 38). However as has been highlighted above, the role of these services and the processes adopted have to change dramatically.

The principles of community development are that change comes from below and the processes are just as important as the outcomes (Ife, 2002). It is not enough to secure user participation in service delivery – that participation has to come about because members of the particular community or group want it, and in ways that they have identified. Clarke (2000, p. 12) argues that the principles of community development are uncompromising: the community identifies the need to change and organisation is through full, voluntary and cooperative efforts of the 'client' population. Hence Ife argues that the outcomes should not be driven or imposed by policy makers or elected members (politicians) but should reflect what the community wants and needs. To achieve this there has to be attention to:

- process and outcomes
- integrity of the process
- participatory democracy
- decentralisation
- accountability
- education
- obligation. (Ife, 2002, p. 119)

But the challenge comes from those individuals and groups who are not necessarily part of, or welcome in, wider communities. Social justice, inclusiveness, anti-discrimination and equal opportunities are core to community development (Barr *et al.*, 1998). However, certain groups with community care needs might challenge communities, either because of how they are perceived, stereotyped and stigmatised, or because the community does not perceive itself as having the capacity to provide the necessary care for individuals and groups. Barr *et al.* (1998) argue that the capacity of service users to define their own needs and seek solutions to their problems is no different from other communities (or others in communities). This is a fundamental principle of personalisation. However, for this to be effective requires 'communities' to be identified and fostered that are not dependent on geographical boundaries but on shared identity and/or shared need. Ferguson and Woodward (2009) argue that it has to involve *collective responses* to *collective problems* (p. 134). For them collective approaches are part of new radical practices that encourage and enable people to link to wider social and political movements. Hence community development can explode myths. The outcome might be not that the community has to provide resources but that service users organise themselves to demand different services or different allocation of resources to ensure that needs are met.

Practice focus

The Positive Mental Attitudes Project at Greater Easterhouse, Glasgow, seeks to address the stigma experienced by people with mental ill health and promote positive attitudes in Greater Easterhouse. It developed from a meeting of Greater Easterhouse Mental Health Forum. The Forum itself came about as a result of threatened closure of services for people with mental health problems. It is a properly constituted organisation led by representatives of mental health users. Local organisations, voluntary and statutory, can be members of the forum, and staff from Health and Social Services are invited to be advisers to the Forum. At an inaugural meeting attended by 80 people, many of whom had mental health problems, stigma was identified as the main problem that needed to be addressed.

A study was therefore set up to assess knowledge and awareness towards mental health attitudes, and identify what training was available. It surveyed employers, service providers, pupils and students at schools and colleges and identified, among other things, lack of awareness of mental health issues, little effort to promote mental health in the work place and lack of training/guidelines on mental health issues.

The Project is user led and user controlled (see Chapter 3), and utilises a community development approach to ascertain the experiences of those who might otherwise be deemed to be service recipients. A centralised top-down approach might have identified the need for day centres or domiciliary care. The identification of stigma as the greatest barrier to those with mental health problems meant activities and resources could be targeted to make a difference and, just as importantly, those resources could draw on the capacities of those who were experiencing the problems.

The Project was funded by Greater Glasgow Health Board and Greater Easterhouse Pathfinder, which aims to encourage and innovate projects in partnership with the local community (see the website for its activities http://www.positivementalattitudes.org.uk/).

Conclusion

This chapter has attempted to give an overview of different approaches to working with communities, and the relationship between this and social work practice. By acknowledging different definitions it has highlighted that policies for working with communities can involve top-down approaches that seek to placate and pacify individuals and groups. Alternative, radical approaches seek to mobilise and motivate. There is a danger that community care policies merely require communities to replace other statutory resources for meeting need. However a community development approach seeks to engage with communities to ensure that needs are identified; resources are demanded and needs are met in ways that are meaningful to those in the community. Such approaches complement and utilise the social work processes associated with advocacy and user empowerment. As such they represent an important context for social work practice.

Point for reflection

There is a lot of discussion in this chapter about definitions of community:

- Think about the 'communities' you are in: geographical, social, educational, etc.
- Now suppose you had a health and/or community care need (in fact you might have one). Where would you want your services – both support services and resources – to come from? To what extent do your various communities feature in helping you meet your needs?

Putting it into practice

A useful way of trying to understand meanings of community is to try to develop a profile of one.

1 Identify a neighbourhood in which you are working. Decide why you have chosen this neighbourhood: is it a council estate? Does it have a particular reputation? Does it have specific problems?
2 Develop a profile of this community, that is, try to describe it and get information about the community. Do this by:
   - walking round the area and observing (for example, age of buildings, characteristics of residents);
   - gathering data (for example, statistics on population) from websites and official documents;
   - talking to people in the community;
   - logging what resources there are (shops, meeting facilities, social services offices);
   - noting such things as how accessible the area is for those with limited mobility;
   - reading local literature to find out what the issues are.

3 On the basis of what you observe/identify/collect/learn, identify what you think are the needs of this community. What do you think the strengths are that would enable the community to meet those needs?

4 If you do not think you can do part 3 of the task, how might you find out these things about the community?

Messages from research

SCDC Mental Health (2010) *Sandyhills Community Mental Health and Well-being Consultation* http://www.positivementalattitudes. org.uk/research-evaluation/.

Quinn, N. and Biggs, H. (2010) 'Creating partnerships to improve community mental health and well-being in an area of high deprivation: lessons from a study with highrise flat residents in east Glasgow', *Journal of Public Mental Health*, 9(4), pp. 16–21.

These two pieces illustrate two different ways of producing research reports. They both report on the same piece of practice – a consultation project undertaken by Positive Mental Attitudes, Glasgow. The first is the final report on a project while the second is the 'academic' version written up for a journal – it is a useful exercise to read them both as they are designed for different 'audiences'.

Further resources

Ferguson, I. and Woodward, R. (2009) *Radical social work in practice.* Bristol: Policy Press.
This text provides an excellent critique of traditional social work practice and of the policies that have underpinned it. It argues for radical approaches which include redefinitions of community and emphasis on collective approaches.

Popple, K. (1995) *Analysing Community Work: its theory and practice.* Buckingham: Open University Press.
A useful text that gives a history of community work and an analysis of the political and practice dimensions.

Stepney, P. and Evans, D. (2000) 'Community social work: towards an integrative model of practice', in Stepney, P. and Ford, D. (eds) *Social Work Models, Methods and Theories.* Lyme Regis: Russell House. This chapter explores the links between community work and social work, using case examples and useful diagrams.

The Scottish Community Development Centre website: http://www.scdc.org.uk/ gives examples of a wide range of approaches to community development.

Conclusion

Writing a conclusion to a text that was first written 20 years ago and is now in its fifth edition seems to be a contradiction! One conclusion is that social work, despite its many challenges, is here to stay. Another could be that social work practice is resistant to change.

Reflecting on the material in this edition and how it has developed from earlier editions the conclusion is that, on the contrary, social work is all about change. This edition illustrates that social work involves:

- Sustaining people through change through the use of interventions, such as counselling, crisis and bereavement work.
- Bringing about change in individuals through interventions as different as insight giving and behaviour modification.
- Bringing about change in circumstances by interventions that are task centred or solution focused.
- Working with people through change in interventions, such as groupwork and community work, advocacy and partnership.

What is also apparent is that social work and the various interventions that social workers use take place in a context of change. Societal and governmental changes influence the behaviour of individuals, the social problems with which they have to cope and responses to them. Technological changes influence not only people's lives but the way that social workers go about their tasks.

Having said that there are some constants and these are represented in Figure 1.1. The five editions of this introduction to social work practice are testimony to the fact that at the centre of all good social work practice is the individual. Also, while the terminology and emphasis might change, social work interventions rely on communications informed by sound values that are committed to the enhancement of the welfare and wellbeing of those individuals.

This fifth edition, therefore, is a continuation of how beginning practitioners can develop understanding and skills – but it remains an introduction. It introduces students and others to the knowledge and contexts of beginning social work practice on which they build as they continue through their professional career. Hopefully, it is also an introduction to the ever-increasing literature and research that is available to enhance their professional practice.

Above all, it is an example of how practice is not an end in itself: by engaging with the wider debates social work will remain a necessary aspect of society. Unfortunately, social problems will never be eradicated but it is to be hoped that the positive contribution that social work interventions can make into the lives of individuals and therefore to society as a whole will be recognised and respected. This will only happen if practitioners continue to develop their practice by increasing their knowledge, improving their skills and responding to the inevitable changes – not with passive acceptance but with professional pride.

References

Adams, R. (1996) *Social Work and Empowerment*. Basingstoke: BASW/Macmillan.

Agnew, A., Manktelow, R., Haynes, T. and Jones, L. (2010) 'Bereavement assessment practice in hospice settings: challenges for palliative care social workers', *British Journal of Social Work*, Advance Access, published 24 May.

Ahmad, W. I. (1990) *Black Perspectives in Social Work*. Birmingham: Venture Press.

Ahmad, W. I. and Atkins, K. (eds) (1996) *'Race' and Community Care*. Buckingham: Open University Press.

Alexander, C., Edwards, R. and Temple, B., with Kanani, U., Zhuang, L., Miah, M. and Sam, A. (2004) *Using Interpreters to Access Services*. York: Joseph Rowntree Foundation.

Allen, G. (1991) 'Social work, community care, and informal networks', in M. Davies (ed.) *Sociological Perspectives on Social Work*. London: Routledge.

Aros-Atolagbe, J. (1990) 'Soapbox', *Social Work Today*, 21(35), p. 36.

Audit Report Commission (1994) *Seen But Not Heard*. London: HMSO.

Ayre, P and Barrett, D. (2003) 'Theory and practice: the chicken and the egg', *European Journal of Social Work*, 6(2), pp. 125–32.

Baginsky, M., Moriarty, J., Manthorpe, J., Stevens, M., MacInnes, T. and Nagendran, T. (2010) *'Social Workers' Workload Survey: Messages from the Frontline. Findings from the 2009 Survey and Interviews with Senior Managers'* (pdf,2,389 KB). London: Department for Children, Schools and Families; Department of Health.

Bailey, R. and Brake, M. (eds) (1975) *Radical Social Work*. London: Edward Arnold.

Bandura, A. (1977) *Social Learning Theory*. Englewood Cliffs, NJ: Prentice-Hall.

Banks, S. (2006) *Ethics and Values in Social Work*, 3rd edn. Basingstoke: Palgrave Macmillan.

Barclay, P. (1982) *Social Workers: their role and tasks*. London: Bedford Square Press.

Barnes, M. (2008) 'Is the personal no longer political?', *Soundings*, 39, pp. 152–9.

Barnes, M. (2011) 'Abandoning Care? A Critical Perspective on Personalisation from an Ethic of Care', *Ethics and Social Welfare*, 5(2), pp. 153–67.

Barr, A., Drysdale, J. *et al.* (1998) 'Raising the potential of community care – the role of community development', *Issues in Social Work Education*, 18(1), pp. 26–46.

Barton, R. (2002) 'The carer's perspective', in M. Davies (ed.) *The Blackwell Companion to Social Work*. Oxford: Blackwell.

Beck, A. T. (1989) *Cognitive Therapy and the Emotional Disorders*. Harmondsworth: Penguin.

Bell, L. (2005) 'Review', in Adams, R., Dominelli, L. and Payne, M. (2002) *Social Work Futures*. Basingstoke: Palgrave Macmillan.

Bell, M. and Wilson, K. (2002) *Practitioner's Guide to Working with Families*. Basingstoke: Palgrave Macmillan.

Benner, P. (1984) *From Novice to Expert: excellence and power in clinical nursing practice*. London: Addison-Wesley.

Beresford, P. (2000) 'Users' knowledges and social work theory: conflict or collaboration?', *British Journal of Social Work*, 30(4), pp. 489–504.

Berger, P. and Luckman, T. (1967) *The Social Construction of Reality: a treatise in the sociology of knowledge*. New York: Doubleday.

Bhatti-Sinclair, K. (2011) *Anti Racist Practice in Social Work*. Basingstoke: Palgrave Macmillan.

Biestek, F. (1957) *The Casework Relationship*. London: Allen & Unwin.

Bowlby, J. (1953) 'Some pathological processes set in train by early mother–child separation', *British Journal of Psychiatry*, 99, pp. 265–72.

Bradshaw, J. (1972) 'A taxonomy of social need', *New Society* (March), 640–3.

Brand, D., Reith, T. and Statham, D. (2005) *The Need for Social Work Intervention: A Discussion paper for the Scottish 21st Century Social Work Review*. http://www.scotland.gov.uk/Publications/2005/12/16105307/53072

Brandon, M., Schofield, G. and Trinder, L. (1998) *Social Work with Children*. Basingstoke: Palgrave Macmillan.

Braye, S. and Preston-Shoot, M. (1995) *Empowering Practice in Social Care*. Buckingham: Open University Press.

British Association for Counselling and Psychotherapy (2011) http://www.itsgoodtotalk.org.uk/search?q=Counselling&x=51&y=8.

Broad, G. (2005) 'Relationship-based practice and reflective practice: holistic approaches to contemporary child care social work', *Child and Family Social Work*, 10, pp. 111–23.

Broadhurst, K., Wastell, D., White, S., Hall, C., Peckover, S., Thompson, K., Pithouse, A. and Davey, D. (2010) 'Performing "initial assessment": identifying the latent conditions for error at the front-door of Local Authority Children's Services', *British Journal of Social Work*, 40(2), pp.352–70.

Brown, A. (1992) *Groupwork*. London: Heinemann l.

Brown, A. (2002) 'Groupwork', in M. Davies (ed.) *Blackwell Companion to Social Work*. Oxford: Blackwell.

Brown, L. (2003) 'Mainstream or margin? The current use of family group conferences in child welfare practice in the UK', *Child and Family Social Work*, 8, 331–40.

Butler, I. and Roberts, G. (2004) *Social Work with Children and Families*. London: Jessica Kingsley.

Bywaters, P. (1975) 'Ending casework relationships', *Social Work Today*, 6(10), pp. 301–4 and 6(11), pp. 336–8.

Calouste Gulbenkian Foundation (1968) *Community Work and Social Change: a report on training*. London: Longman.

Cambridge, P. and Forrester-Jones, R. (2003) 'Using individualised communication for interviewing people with intellectual disability: a case study of user-centred research', *Journal of Intellectual & Developmental Disability*, 28(1), pp. 5–23.

Canton, R. (2005) 'Risk assessment and compliance in probation and mental health practice', in Littlechild, B. and Feams, D. (eds) *Mental Disorder and Criminal Justice: policy, provision and practice*. Lyme Regis: Russell House.

Caplan, G. (1964) *Principles of Preventive Psychiatry*. London: Tavistock.

Carpenter, J. and Schneider, J. (2004) 'Integration and targeting of community care for people with severe and enduring mental health problems: users' experiences of the care programme approach and care management', *British Journal of Social Work*, 34(3), pp. 313–14.

Carr, S. (2010) *Personalisation: a rough guide (revised edition)* Scie Report no. 20 London, SCIE http://www.scie.org.uk/publications/reports/report20.pdf.

Cavanagh, K. and Cree, V. E. (eds) (1996) *Working With Men: feminism and social work*. London: Routledge.

CCETSW/IAMHW (1989) *Multidisciplinary Teamwork: models of good practice*. London: Central Council for Education and Training in Social Work.

Challis, D., Chessum, R., Chesterman, J., Luckett, R. and Traske, K. (1990) *Case Management in Social and Health Care*. Canterbury: Personal Social Services Research Unit.

Chaplin, J. (1988) *Feminist Counselling in Action*. London: Sage.

Charnley, H. M. and Langley, J. (2007) 'Developing cultural competence as a framework for anti-heterosexist social work practice: reflections from the UK', *Journal of Social Work*, 7, pp. 307–21.

Christie, A. (2001) *Men and Social Work: theories and practices*. Basingstoke: Palgrave Macmillan.

Clarke, S. (2000) *Social Work as Community Development*. Aldershot: Ashgate.

Cleaver, H. and Walker, S. (2004) 'From policy to practice: the implementation of a new framework for social work assessments of children and families', *Child and Family Social Work*, 9, pp. 81–90.

Cleaver, H., Steve Walker, S., Scott, J., Cleaver, D., Rose, W., Ward, H. and Pithouse, A. (2008) *The Integrated Children's System Enhancing Social Work and Inter-Agency Practice*, London. Jessica Kingsley.

Clifford, D. and Burke, B. (2009) *Anti-Oppressive Ethics and Values in Social Work*. Basingstoke: Palgrave Macmillan.

Cohen, M. and Mullender, A. (eds) (2003) *Gender and Group-work*. London: Routledge.

Colton, M., Sanders, B. and Williams, C. (2001) *An Introduction to Working with Children*. Basingstoke: Palgrave Macmillan.

Coote, A. (ed.) (1992) *The Welfare of Citizens*. London: Institute for Public Policy Research/Rivers Oram Press.

Corby, B. (1996) 'Risk assessment in child protection work', in Kemshall, H. and Pritchard, J. (eds) *Good Practice in Risk Assessment and Risk Management*. London: Jessica Kingsley.

Corcoran, J. and Pillai, V. (2009) 'A review of research on solution-focused therapy', *British Journal of Social Work*, 39(2), pp. 234–42.

Cossis-Brown, H. (2008) 'Social work and sexuality: working with lesbians and gay men: what remains the same and what is Different?', *Practice*, 20(4), pp. 265–75.

Coulshed, V. (1991) *Social Work Practice: an introduction*. Basingstoke: BASW/Macmillan.

Coulshed, V. and Orme, J. (2006) *Social Work Practice*, 4th edn, Basingstoke: Palgrave Macmillan.

Cree, V. and Sidhva, D. (2011) 'Children and HIV in Scotland: findings from a cross-sector needs assessment of children and young people infected and affected by HIV in Scotland', *British Journal of Social Work*, Advance Access, published 5 April.

Cree, V. and Myers, S. (2008) *Social Work Making a Difference*. Bristol: Policy Press/BASW.

Currer, C. (2002) 'Dying and bereavement', in Adams, R., Dominelli, L. and Payne, M. (eds) *Critical Practice in Social Work*. Basingstoke: Palgrave Macmillan.

Dalrymple, J. and Burke, B. (1995) *Anti-Oppressive Practice: social care and the law*. Buckingham: Open University Press.

Daniel, B. and Wassell, S. (2002) *Assessing and Promoting Resilience in Vulnerable Children 1: Early years*. London: Jessica Kingsley.

Davies, M. (1985) *The Essential Social Worker: a guide to positive practice*. Aldershot: Wildwood House.

Day, A., O'Leary, P., Chung, D. and Justo, D. (2009) *Integrated Responses to Domestic Violence: Research and Practice Experiences in Working with Men*. Annandale NSW: Federation Press (Willan Publishing in the UK).

DCSF (2009) Building a Safe Confident Future: the final report of the Social Work Task Force, London, DCSF.

de Shazer, S. (1988) *Clues: investigating solutions in brief therapy*. New York and London: Norton.

de Zuluetta, F. (2010) 'Reflective practice using attachment therapy', in Webber, M. and Nathan, J. (eds) *Reflective Practice in Mental Health*. London: Jessica Kingsley.

Department for Education (2010) *The Munro Review of Child Protection Interim Report: The Children's Journey*. London: HMSO.

Department for Education (2011) *The Munro Review of Child Protection: Final Report – A child-centred system*. London: HMSO.

Department of Health, Cmnd 849 (1989) *Caring for People: community care in the next decade and beyond*. London: HMSO.

Department of Health/Social Services Inspectorate (SSI) (1989b) *Homes are for Living In*. London: HMSO.

Department of Health Social Services/SSI and Scottish Office Social Work Services Group (1991) *Care Management and Assessment: practitioner's guide*. London: HMSO.

Department of Health (1995) *Child Protection: messages from research*. London: HMSO.

Department of Health (1996) *Refocusing Children's Services*. London: HMSO.

Department of Health (2000a) *A Practitioner's Guide to Carers' Assessments under the Carers and Disabled Children Act*. London: DoH.

Department of Health (2000b) *The NHS Plan: a plan for investment, a plan to reform*. London: DoH.

Department of Health (2000c) *Framework for Assessment of Children in Need and their Families*. London: DoH

Department of Health (2001) *The National Service Framework for Older People*. London: DoH.

Department of Health (2002a) *The Single Assessment Process: Guidance for Local Implementation*. London: DoH.

Department of Health (2002b) *Fair Access to Care Services*. London: DoH.

Department of Health (2005) 'Delivering race equality in mental health care: an action plan for reform inside and outside services', London: DoH.

Department of Health (2008a) *Evaluation of the New Social Work Degree Qualification in England. Volume 1: Findings*. London, Social Care Workforce Research Unit, King's College London, http://www.dh.gov.uk/prod_consum_dh/group.

Department of Health (2008b) *Local Government Circular LAC (DH) (2008) 1: Transforming Social Care*, London, DoH.

Doel, M. (2002) 'Task centred practice', in Adams, R., Dominelli, L. and Payne, M. (eds) *Social Work: themes issues and critical debates*. Basingstoke: Palgrave Macmillan.

Doel, M. and Sawdon, C. (1999) *The Essential Groupwork: teaching and learning creative groupwork*. London: Jessica Kingsley.

Doel, M. and Sawdon, C. (2001) 'What makes for successful groupwork? A survey of agencies in the UK', *British Journal of Social Work*, 31(3), pp. 437–63.

Dominelli, L. (1988) *Antiracist Social Work*. Basingstoke: Macmillan.

Dominelli, L. (2000) 'Empowerment: help or hindrance in professional relationships', in Stepney, P. and Ford, D. (eds) *Social Work Models Methods and Theories: a framework for practice*. Lyme Regis: Russell House Publishing.

Dominelli, L. (2002a) *Feminist Social Work Theory and Practice*, Basingstoke: Palgrave Macmillan.

Dominelli, L. (2002b) *Anti-Oppressive Social Work Theory and Practice* Basingstoke: Palgrave Macmillan.

Dominelli, L. and McLeod, E. (1989) *Feminist Social Work*. Basingstoke: Macmillan.

Doyal, L. (1993) 'Human need and the moral right to optimal community care', in Bornat, J., Johnson, J., Pereira, C., Pilgrim, D. and Williams, F. (eds) *Community Care: a reader*. Buckingham: Open University/Macmillan.

Doyal, L. and Gough, I. (1991) *A Theory of Human Need*. Basingstoke: Macmillan.

Egan, G. (1981) *The Skilled Helper: a model for systematic helping and interpersonal relating*. California: Brooks/Cole.

Eichenbaum, L. and Orbach, S. (1983) *Understanding Women*. Harmondsworth: Penguin.

Ellis, A. (1962) *Reason and Emotion in Psychotherapy*. New York: Lyle Stuart.

Ellis, K. (2007) 'Direct payments and social work practice: the significance of "street-level bureaucracy" in determining eligibility', *British Journal of Social Work*, 37(3), pp. 405–22.

England, H. (1986) *Social Work as Art: making sense for good practice*. London: Allen & Unwin.

Erikson, E. (1965) *Childhood and Society*. Harmondsworth: Penguin.

Evans, R. (1976) 'Some implications of an integrated model for social work theory and practice', *British Journal of Social Work*, 6(2), pp. 177–200.

Fawcett, B. (2010) *Postmodernism*, in Gray, M. and S. Webb (eds) *Social Work Theories and Methods*. London: Sage.

Featherstone, B. (1997) ' "I wouldn't do your job!" Women, social work and child abuse', in Hollway, W. and Featherstone, B. (eds) *Mothering and Ambivalence*. London: Routledge.

Featherstone, B. (2003) 'Taking fathers seriously', *British Journal of Social Work*, 33, pp. 239–54.

Featherstone, B. (2004) *Family Life and Support: a feminist analysis*. Basingstoke: Palgrave Macmillan.

Featherstone, B. (2006a) 'Rethinking family support in the current policy context', *British Journal of Social Work* 36, 5–19

Featherstone (2006b) 'Why gender matters in child welfare and protection', *Critical Social Policy* Special Issue, 26(2), 294–315.

Featherstone, B. and Fawcett, B. (1995) '"Oh no! Not more isms!"', *Social Work Education*, 14(3), pp. 25–43.

Ferguson, I. and Woodward, R. (2009) *Radical Social Work in Practice: Making a Difference*. Bristol: Policy Press.

Fischer, J. (1976) 'Older male carers and community care', in Bornat, J. Johnson, J., Pereira, C., Pilgrim, D. and Williams, F. (eds) *Community Care: a reader*. Buckingham: Open University/Macmillan.

Fook, J. (2002) *Social Work Critical Theory and Practice*. London: Routledge.

Fook, J. and Askeland, G. (2007) 'Challenges of critical reflection: "nothing ventured, nothing gained"', *Social Work Education the International Journal*, 26(5), pp. 520–33.

Fook, J. and Gardner, F. (2007) *Practising Critical Reflection: a resource handbook*. Maidenhead: Open University Press.

Fook, J., Ryan, M. and Hawkins. L. (2000) *Professional Expertise: practice, theory and education for working in uncertainty*. London: Whiting & Birch.

Ford, P. and Postle, K. (2001) 'Task-centred practice and care management', in Stepney, P. and Ford, D. (eds) *Social Work Models, Methods and Theories*. Lyme Regis: Russell House.

Forrester, D., McCambridge, M., Waissbein, C., Emlyn-Jones, R. and Rollnick, S. (2008) 'Child risk and parental resistance: can motivational interviewing improve the practice of child and family social workers in working with parental alcohol misuse?', *British Journal of Social Work*, 38(7), pp. 1302–19.

Freire, P. (1972) *Pedagogy of the Oppressed*. Harmondsworth: Penguin.

Froggett, L. (2000) 'The supervision of social workers', in Davies, M. (ed.) *The Blackwell Encyclopaedia of Social Work*. Oxford: Blackwell.

Frost, N., Jefferys, L. and Lloyd, A. (2003) *The RHP Companion to Family Support*. Lyme Regis: Russell House.

Garrett, A. (1972) *Interviewing: its Principles and Methods*. New York: Family Service Association of America.

Garrett, P. (2003) 'Swimming with the dolphins: the new assessment framework, New Labour and new tools for social work with children and families', *British Journal of Social Work*, 33(4), pp. 441–64.

Gibbons, J. S., Bow, I., Butler, J. and Powell, J. (1979) 'Clients' reaction to task-centred casework: a follow-up study', *British Journal of Social Work*, 9(2), pp. 203–15.

Gilligan, R. (1998) 'Beyond permanence? The importance of resilience in child placement and planning', in Hill, M. and Shaw, M. (eds) *Signposts in Adoption: Policy, practice and research issues*. London: BAAF.

Goldberg, E. M., Gibbons, J. and Sinclair, I. (1985) *Problems, Tasks and Outcomes: the evaluation of task-centred casework in three settings.* London: George Allen & Unwin.

Goldberg, E. M., Walker, D. and Robinson, J. (1977) 'Exploring the task-centred casework method', *Social Work Today*, 9(2), pp. 9–14.

Goldstein, H. (1973) *Social Work Practice: a unitary approach.* Columbia, SC: University of South Carolina Press.

Golembiewski, R. T. and Blumberg, A. (eds) (1970) *Sensitivity Training and the Laboratory Approach.* Itasca, IL: Peacock.

Gorman, K. (2001) 'Cognitive behaviourism and the holy grail: the quest for a universal means of managing offender risk', *Probation Journal*, 48(3), pp. 3–9.

Gorman, H. and Postle, K. (2003) *Transforming Community Care: a distorted vision?* Birmingham: Venture Press.

Gorrell Barnes, G. (1984) *Working with Families.* London: Macmillan.

Hafford-Letchfield, T. (2007) *Practicing Quality Assurance in Social Care.* Exeter: Learning Matters.

Healy, K. (2005) *Social Work Theories in Context*, Basingstoke: Palgrave Macmillan.

Heap, K. (1985) *The Practice of Social Work with Groups: a systematic approach.* London: George Allen & Unwin.

Henderson, P. and Thomas, D.N. (1981) *Skills in Neighbourhood Work.* London: George Allen & Unwin.

Hester, M. and Radford, J. (1996) 'Contradictions and compromises: the impact of the Children Act on women and children's safety', in Hester, M., Kelley, L. and Radford, J. (eds) *Women, Violence and Male Power.* Buckingham: Open University Press.

Hill, M. (1999) *Effective Ways of Working with Children and their Families.* London: Jessica Kingsley.

Hill, M. (2002) 'Network assessments and diagrams: a flexible friend in social work and education', *Journal of Social Work*, 2(2), pp. 233–54.

Hodgkinson, P. and Stewart, M. (1991) *Coping with Catastrophe: a professional handbook for post-disaster aftercare.* London: Routledge.

Hogg, V. and Wheeler, J. (2004) 'Miracles R them: solution-focused practice in a Social Services Duty Team', *Practice*, 16(4).

Hollis, F. (1964) *Casework: a psychosocial therapy.* New York: Random House.

Hollis, F. (1970) 'The psychosocial approach to the practice of casework', in Roberts, R.W. and. Nee, R.H. (eds) *Theories of Social Casework.* Chicago: University of Chicago Press.

Holman, B. (1998) 'From children's departments to family departments', *Child and Family Social Work*, 3, pp. 205–11.

Hong Chui, W. and Ford, D. (2000) 'Crisis intervention as common practice', in Stepney, P. and Ford, D. (eds) *Social Work Models Methods and Theories: a framework for practice.* Lyme Regis: Russell House.

Horder, W. (2002) 'Care management', in Davies, M. (ed.) *The Blackwell Companion to Social Work*. Oxford: Blackwell.

Houston, S. (2002) 'Re-thinking a systematic approach to child welfare: a critical response to the framework for the assessment of children in need and their families', *European Journal of Social Work*, 5(3), pp. 301–12.

Howe, D. (1987) *An Introduction to Social Work Theory*. Aldershot: Community Care Practice Handbooks.

Howe, D. (1992) *An Introduction to Social Work Theory: making sense in practice*, 3rd edn. Aldershot: Wildwood House.

Howe, D. (1994) 'Modernity, postmodernity and social work', *British Journal of Social Work*, 24(5), pp. 513–32.

Howe, D. (1995) *Attachment Theory for Social Work Practice*. London: Macmillan.

Howe, D. (1997) 'Psychosocial relationship-based theories for child and family social work: political philosophy, psychology and welfare practice', *Child and Family Social Work*, 2(3), pp. 161–9.

Howe, D. (2000) 'Relating theory to practice', in Davies, M. (ed.) *Blackwell Companion to Social Work*. Oxford: Blackwell.

Howe, D. (2006) 'Disabled children, parent–child interaction and attachment', *Child and and Family Social Work*, 11(2), pp. 95–106.

Howe, D. and Fearnley, S. (2003) 'Disorders of attachment in adopted and fostered children: recognition and treatment', *Clinical Child Psychology and Psychiatry*, 8 (3), pp. 369–87.

Hudson, B. L. and Macdonald, G. M. (1986) *Behavioural Social Work: an introduction*. London: Macmillan.

Ife, J. (2002) *Community Development: Community based alternatives in an age of globalisation*. Frenchs Forest NSW: Longman.

Iveson, C. (2002) 'Solution-focused brief therapy', *Advances in Psychiatric Treatment*, 8(2), pp. 149–57.

Jack, G. and Jack, D. (2000) 'Ecological social work: the application of a systems model of development in context', in Stepney, P. and Ford, D. (eds) *Social Work Models, Methods and Theories*. Lyme Regis: Russell House.

Jehu, E (1967) *Learning Theory and Social Work*. London: Routledge & Kegan Paul.

Jones, C. (1996) 'Anti-intellectualism and the peculiarities of British social work education', in Parton, N. (ed.) *Social Theory, Social Change and Social Work*. London: Routledge.

Jordan, B. (1972) *The Social Worker in Family Situations*. London: Routledge & Kegan Paul.

Kadushin, A. (1972) *The Social Work Interview*. New York: Columbia University Press.

Keating, F. (2000) 'Anti-racist perspectives: what are the gains?', *Social Work Education*, 19(1), pp. 76–87.

Kelly, G. A. (1955) *The Psychology of Personal Constructs*. New York: Norton.

Kemshall, H. (2002) 'Risk, public protection and justice', in Ward, D. Scott, J. and Lacey, M. (eds) *Probation: Working for Justice*, 2nd edn, pp. 95–109. Oxford: Oxford University Press.

Kemshall, H. and Littlechild, R. (eds) (2000) *User Involvement and Participation in Social Care: research informing practice*. London: Jessica Kingsley.

Kenny, L. and Kenny, B. (2000) 'Psychodynamic theory in social work: a view from practice', in Stepney, P. and Ford, D. (eds) *Social Work Models, Methods and Theories*. Lyme Regis: Russell House.

Lancaster, E. and Lumb, J. (2006) 'The assessment of risk in the National Probation Service of England and Wales', *Journal of Social Work*, 6, pp. 275–91.

Lask, J. (2010) 'Reflective practice using systemic family therapy', in Webber, M. and Nathan, J. (eds) *Reflective Practice in Mental Health*. London: Jessica Kingsley.

Lawton, A. (2007) *Supporting Self-advocacy* Scie position paper 6. London: Scie http://www.scie.org.uk/publications/positionpapers/pp06.asp.

Leadbetter, M. (2002) 'Empowerment and advocacy', in Adams, R., Dominelli, L. and Payne, M. (eds) *Social Work Themes: issues and critical debates*. Basingstoke: Palgrave Macmillan.

Lefevre, M. (2010) *Communicating with Children and Young People Making a Difference*. Bristol: Policy Press.

Lindemann, E. (1965) 'Symptomatology and management of acute grief', in Parad, H.J. (ed.) *Crisis Interventions: selected readings*. New York: Family Service Association of America.

Linehan, M. M. (1987) 'Dialectical behavior therapy: a cognitive behavioral approach to parasuicide', *Journal of Personality Disorders*, 1, 328–33.

Lishman, J. (1995) *Communication in Social Work*. Basingstoke: BASW/Macmillan.

Littlechild, B. and Hawley, C. (2010) 'Risk assessment for mental health service users: ethical, valid and reliable?', *Journal of Social Work*, 10, pp. 211–29.

Loney, M. (1983) *Community Against Government*. London: Heinemann.

Lupton, C. (1998) 'User empowerment or family self-reliance? The family group conference model', *British Journal of Social Work*, 28(1), pp. 107–28.

Lynch, R. and Garrett, P.M. (2010) ' "More than words": touch practices in child and family social work', *Child & Family Social Work*, 15(4), pp. 389–98.

Macrae, R. and Andrews, M. (2000) 'Work with men who abuse women partners', *Probation Journal*, 47(1), pp. 30–8.

Marsh, P. (2002) 'Task centred work', in Davies, M. (ed.) *Blackwell Companion to Social Work*. Oxford: Blackwell.

Marsh, P. and Doel, M. (2005) *The Task-centred Book*. London: Routledge.

Marsh, P. and Fisher, M. (1992) *Good Intentions: partnership in social services*. York: Joseph Rowntree Foundation.

Maslow, A. (1954) *Motivation and Personality*, 2nd edn. New York:Harper & Row.

Mayer, J. E. and Timms, N. (1970) *The Client Speaks: working class impressions of casework*. London: Routledge & Kegan Paul.

Mayo, M. (1994) 'Community work', in Hanvey, C. and Philpot, T. (eds) *Practising Social Work*. London: Routledge.

Mayo, M. (2002) 'Community work', in Adams, R., Dominelli, L. and Payne, M. (eds) *Social Work: themes, issues and critical debates*. Basingstoke: Palgrave Macmillan.

McLaughlin, H. (2009) 'What's in a name: "client", "patient", "customer", "consumer", "expert by experience", "service user" – what's next?', *British Journal of Social Work*, 39, pp. 1101–17.

McGuire, J. (ed.) (1995) *What Works: reducing re-offending*. Chichester: Wiley.

McNeill, F. (2000) 'Making criminology work: theory and practice in local context', *Probation Journal*, 47(2), pp. 108–18.

McNeill, F., Batchelor, S., Burnett, R. and Know, J. (2005) *21st Century Social Work*. Edinburgh: Scottish Executive.

McNeill, F. and B. Whyte (2007) *Reducing Reoffending: Social Work and Community Justice in Scotland*. Portland, Willan.

Means, R., Richards, S. and Smith, R. (2003) *Community Care: policy and practice*, 3rd edn. Basingstoke: Macmillan.

Mearns, D. and Thorne, B. (1998) *Person-centred Counselling in Action*. London: Sage.

Milner, J. (2000) 'Solution focused therapy', in Davies, M. (ed.) *The Blackwell Encyclopaedia of Social Work*. Oxford: Blackwell.

Milner, J. (2001) *Women and Social Work: narrative approaches*. Basingstoke: Palgrave Macmillan.

Milner, J. and O'Byrne, P. (2002) *Assessment in Social Work*. Basingstoke: Palgrave Macmillan.

Minuchin, S. 1974) *Families and Family Therapy*. London: Tavistock.

Mitchell, J. (1984) *Women: the Longest Revolution: essays in feminism literature and psychoanalysis*. London: Virgo.

Morris, J. (1993) 'Feminism and disability', *Feminist Review*, 43, pp. 57–70.

Mullender, A. (1996) *Rethinking Domestic Violence: the social work and probation response*. London: Routledge.

Mullender, A. and Morley, R. (eds) (1994) *Children Living with Domestic Violence: putting men's abuse of women on the child care agenda*. London: Whiting & Birch.

Mullender, A. and Ward, D. (1991) *Self-Directed Groupwork: users take action for empowerment*. London: Whiting & Birch.

Munn-Giddings, C. and McVicar, A. (2007) 'Self-help groups as mutual support: what do carers value?', *Health & Social Care in the Community*, 15(1), pp. 26–34.

Myers, S. (2007) *Solution Focused Approaches*. Lyme Regis: Russell House Press.

Newbigging K. and Thomas, N. with Coupe, J., Habte-Mariam, Z., Ahmed, N., Shah, A. and Hicks, J. (2010) *Good Practice in Social Care for Refugees and Asylum Seekers*, Scie Report 31, London: Scie.

Newburn, T. (ed.) (1996) *Working with Disaster: social welfare interventions during and after tragedy*. Harlow: Longman.

Northen, H. (1969) *Social Work with Groups*. New York: Colombia University Press.

Nuttman-Shwartz, O., Dekel, R. and. Tuval-Mashiach, R. (2010) 'Post-traumatic stress and growth following forced relocation', *British Journal of Social Work*, Advance Access, published 15 November.

O'Connell, B. (2004) *Solution Focused Therapy*. London: Sage.

O'Hagan, K. (1986) *Crisis Intervention in Social Services*. London: Macmillan.

Oliver, M. (1996) *Understanding Disability: from theory to practice*. Basingstoke: Macmillan.

Orme, J. (1995) *Workloads: measurement and management*. Aldershot: Avebury (in association with CEDR).

Orme, J. (2000a) 'Social work: "the appliance of social science" – a cautionary tale', *Journal of Social Work Education*, 19(4), pp. 323–34.

Orme, J. (2000b) 'Interactive social sciences: patronage or partnership', *Science and Public Policy*, 27(3), pp. 211–19.

Orme, J. (2001a) *Gender and Community Care: social work and social care perspectives*. Basingstoke: Palgrave Macmillan.

Orme, J. (2001b) 'Regulation or fragmentation? Directions for social work under New Labour', *British Journal of Social Work*, 31, pp. 611–24.

Orme, J. (2002a) 'Feminist social work', in Adams, R. Dominelli, L. and Payne, M. (eds) *Social Work Themes, Issues and Critical Debates*, 2nd edn. Basingstoke: Palgrave Macmillan.

Orme, J. (2002b) 'Social work: gender, care and justice', *British Journal of Social Work*, 32(6), pp. 799–814.

Orme, J. (2009) 'Feminist social work', in Gray, M. and Webb, S.A. (eds) *Social Work: Theories and Methods*. London: Sage.

Orme, J. and Glastonbury, B. (1993) *Care Management*. Basingstoke: BASW/Macmillan.

Orme, J. and Shemmings, D. (2010) *Developing Research Based Social Work Practice*. Basingstoke: Palgrave Macmillan.

Orme, J., Dominelli, L. and Mullender, A. (2000) 'Working with violent men from a feminist perspective', *International Social Work*, 43(1), pp. 89–108.

O'Sullivan T. (1999) *Decision-making in Social Work*. Basingstoke: Macmillan.

Papell, C. P. and Rothman, B. (1966) 'Social groupwork models: possession and heritage', *Journal of Education for Social Work*, 2(2), pp. 66–77.

Parad, H. J. and Caplan, G. (1965) 'A framework for studying families in crisis', in Parad, H.J. (ed.) *Crisis Intervention: selected readings*. New York: Family Service Association of America.

Parker, J. and Bradley, G. (2003) *Social Work Practice: assessment, planning, intervention and review*. Exeter: Learning Matters.

Parkes, C. M. (1986) *Bereavement: studies of grief in adult life*. London: Tavistock.

Parry, G. (1990) *Coping with Crises*. Leicester: British Psychological Society/Routledge.

Parton, N. (1998) 'Risk, advanced liberalism and child welfare: the need to rediscover uncertainty and ambiguity', *British Journal of Social Work*, 28(1), pp. 5–27.

Parton, N. (2000) 'Some thoughts on the relationship between theory and practice in and for social work', *British Journal of Social Work*, 30, pp. 449–63.

Parton, N. (2008) 'Changes in the form of knowledge in social work: from the "social" to the "informational"?', *British Journal of Social Work*, 38, pp. 253–69.

Parton, N. and O'Byrne, P. (2000) *Constructive Social Work: towards a new practice*. Basingstoke: Palgrave.

Payne, M. (1986) *Social Care in the Community*. Basingstoke: Macmillan.

Payne, M. (1995) *Social Work and Community Care*. Basingstoke: Macmillan.

Payne, M. (1997) *Modern Social Work Theory: a critical introduction*. Basingstoke: Macmillan.

Payne, M. (1998) 'Social work theories and critical practice', in Adams, R., Dominelli, L. and Payne, M. (eds) *Social Work: themes, issues and critical debates*. Basingstoke: Palgrave Macmillan.

Payne, M. (2000) *Narrative Therapy: an introduction for counsellors*. London: Sage.

Payne, M. (2005) *Modern Social Work Theory: a critical introduction*, 3rd edn. Basingstoke: Palgrave.

Pease, B. and Fook, J. (eds) (1999) *Transforming Social Work Practice: postmodern critical perspectives*. London: Routledge.

Perlman, H. H. (1957) *Social Casework: a problem-solving process*. London: Tavistock/Routledge.

Petch, A. (2002) 'Work with adult service users', in Davies, M. (ed.) *Blackwell Companion to Social Work*. Oxford: Blackwell.

Phillips, J., Mo Ray, M. and Marshall, M. (2006) *Social Work with Older People*, 4th edn. Basingstoke: Palgrave Macmillan.

Pilalis, J. (1986) 'The integration of theory and practice: a re-examination of a paradoxical expectation', *British Journal of Social Work*, 16(1), pp. 79–96.

Pincus, A. and Minahan, A. (1973) *Social Work Practice: model and method*. Itasca, IL: Peacock.

Plant, R. (1973) *Social and Moral Theory in Casework*. London: Routledge & Kegan Paul.

Popple, K. (1995) *Analysing Community Work: its theory and practice*. Buckingham: Open University Press.

Popple, K. (2002) 'Community work', in Adams, R., Dominelli, L. and Payne, M. (eds) *Critical Practice in Social Work*. Basingstoke: Palgrave Macmillan.

Postle, K. (2001) 'The social work side is disappearing. It started with us being called care managers', *Practice*, 13(1), pp. 13–26.

Postle, K. (2002) 'Working "between the idea and the reality": ambiguities and tensions in care managers' work', *British Journal of Social Work*, 32(3), pp. 335–51.

Preston-Shoot, M. (2007) *Effective Groupwork*, 2nd edn. Basingstoke: Palgrave Macmillan.

Prevatt Goldstein, B. (2002) 'Black perspectives', in Davies, M. (ed.) *Blackwell Companion to Social Work*. Oxford: Blackwell.

Prochaska, J. O. and DiClemente, C. (1984) *The Transtheoretical Approach: crossing the traditional boundaries of therapy*. Homewood, IL: Dow Jones/Irwin.

Raphael, B. (1984) *The Anatomy of Bereavement: a handbook for the caring professions*. London: Unwin Hyman.

Raphael, B. (1986) *When Disaster Strikes: a handbook for the caring professions*. London: Hutchinson.

Rapoport, L. (1970) 'Crisis intervention as a brief mode of treatment', in Roberts, R.W. and Nee, R.H. (eds) *Theories of Social Casework*. Chicago: University of Chicago Press.

Reid, W. J. (1978) *The Task-Centred System*. New York: Colombia University Press.

Reid, W. J. and Epstein, L. (1972) *Task-Centred Casework*. New York: Colombia University Press.

Reid, W. J. and Epstein, L. (eds) (1977) *Task-Centred Practice*. New York: Colombia University Press.

Reid, W. J. and Hanrahan, P. (1981) 'The effectiveness of social work: recent evidence', in Goldberg, E.M. and Connolly, N. (eds) *Evaluative Research in Social Care*. London: Heinemann.

Reid, W. J. and Shyne, A. W. (1969) *Brief and Extended Casework*. New York: Colombia University Press.

Remington, B. and Barron, C. (1991) 'Working with problem drinkers: a cognitive behavioural approach', *Probation Journal*, 38(1), pp. 15–19.

Richards, S. (2000) 'Bridging the divide: elders and the assessment process', *British Journal of Social Work*, 30(1), pp. 37–50.

Richmond, M. (1922) *What is Social Case Work?* New York: Russell Sage.

Robinson, L. (1998) *Race: communication and the caring professions*. Buckingham: Open University Press.

Robson, P., Begum, N. *et al.* (2003) *Increasing User Involvement in Voluntary Organisations*. York: Joseph Rowntree Foundation.

Rogers, C. (1980) *A Way of Being*. Boston, MA: Houghton Mifflin.

Rojek, C. (1986) 'The "subject" in social work', *British Journal of Social Work*, 16(1), pp. 65–77.

Rothman, J. (1968) 'Three models of community organization practice their mixing and phasing', in Cox, F.M. *et al.* (eds) *Strategies for Community Organization*, 3rd edn. Itasca, IL: Peacock.

Sainsbury, E. (1975) *Social Work and families: perceptions of social casework among clients of a Family Service Unit*. London, Routledge & Kegan Paul.

Saleeby, D. (1996) 'Strengths perspective in social work practice: extensions and cautions', *Social Work*, 41, pp. 296–305.

Sapey, B. (2004) 'Impairment, disability, and loss: reassessing the rejection of loss', *Illness, Crisis & Loss*, 12(1), pp. 90–101.

Schon, D. A. (1987) *Education and the Reflective Practitioner: toward a new design for teaching and learning in the professions*. California: Jossey-Bass.

Schutz, W. C. (1966) *FIRO: the interpersonal underworld*. New York: Science and Behaviour Books.

Scie (2004) *Teaching and Learning Communication Skills in Social Work Education*. London: Social Care Institute for Excellence.

Scie (2010) *Good Practice in Social Care for Refugees and Asylum Seekers Good Practice Guide*, 26. London: Scie, http://www.scie.org.uk/publications/ataglance/ataglance26.asp.

Scottish Executive (2000) *Community Care: a joint future, Report of the Joint Future Group*. Edinburgh: Scottish Executive.

Scottish Executive (2006a) *Changing Lives: Report of the 21st century Social Work Review*. Edinburgh: Scottish Executive.

Scottish Government (2006b) *The Same As You? A review of services for people with learning disabilities*. Edinburgh: Scottish Government, http://www.dgcommunity.net/dgcommunity/xdocuments/6823.pdf.ashx.

Scottish Government (2008) *Getting it Right for Every Child*. Edinburgh: Scottish Government, http://www.scotland.gov.uk/Topics/People/Young-People/childrensservices/girfec/CoreComponents.

Scourfield, J. (2002) *Gender and Child Protection*. Basingstoke: Palgrave Macmillan.

Scourfield, J. and Coffey, A. (2002) 'Understanding gendered practice in child protection', *Qualitative Social Work*, 1(3), pp. 319–40.

Seden, J. (2005) *Counselling Skills in Social Work Practice*, 2nd edn. Buckingham: Open University Press.

Shaw, I. and Shaw, A. (1997) 'Keeping social work honest: evaluating as profession and practice', *British Journal of Social Work*, 27, pp. 847–69.

Sheldon, B. (1983) 'The use of single-case experimental designs in the evaluation of social work', *British Journal of Social Work*, 13(5), pp. 477–500.

Sheldon, B. (1984) 'Behavioural approaches with psychiatric patients', in M. R. Olsen (ed.) *Social Work and Mental Health*. London: Tavistock.

Sheldon, B. (2000) 'Cognitive behavioural methods in social care: a look at the evidence', in Stepney, P. and. Ford, D. (eds) *Social Work Models, Methods and Theories*. Lyme Regis: Russell House.

Sheldon, B. and Chilvers, R. (2001) *Evidence-based Social Care: A study of prospects and problems*. Lyme Regis: Russell House.

Sheldon, F. (1997) *Psychosocial Palliative Care*. Cheltenham: Stanley Thornes.

Shemmings, D. (2004) 'Researching relationships from an attachment perspective: the use of behavioural, interview, self report and projective measures', *Journal of Social Work Practice*, 18(3), pp. 299–314.

Silverman, P.R. (2004) 'Bereavement: a time of transition and changing relationships', in Berzoff, J. and Silverman, P.R. (eds) *Living with Dying: A handbook for end-of-life healthcare practitioners*. New York: Columbia University Press.

Siporin, M. (1975) *Introduction to Social Work Practice*. New York: Macmillan.

Skinner, B. F. (1938) *The Behaviour of Organisms*. New York: Appleton.

Smale, G., Tuson, G., Cooper, M., Wardle, M. and Crosbie, D. (1988) *Community Social Work: a paradigm for change*. London: NISW.

Smale, G., Tuson, G., Biehal, N. and Marsh, P. (1993) *Empowerment, Assessment, Care Management and the Skilled Worker*, National Institute for Social Work Practice and Development Exchange. London: HMSO.

Smith, D. (2005) 'Probation and social work', *British Journal of Social Work*, 35, pp. 621–37.

Smith, D. and Vanstone, M. (2002) 'Probation and social justice', *British Journal of Social Work*, 32(6), pp. 815–31.

Smith, M. (2009) *Rethinking Residential Childcare*. Bristol: Policy Press.

Smith, P. B. (1980) *Group Processes and Personal Change*. London and Cambridge, MA: Harper & Row.

Specht, H. and Vickery, A. (eds) (1977) *Integrating Social Work Methods*. London: Allen & Unwin.

Stanley, L. and Wise, S. (1990) *Feminist Praxis: research, theory and epistemology in feminist sociology*. London: Routledge.

Stepney, P. and Ford, D. (eds) (2000) *Social Work Models, Methods and Theories*. Lyme Regis: Russell House.

Stuart, O. (1996) ' "Yes, we mean black disabled people too": thoughts on community care and disabled people from black and minority ethnic communities', in Ahmad, W.U.I. and Atkin, K. (eds) *'Race' and Community Care*. Buckingham: Open University Press.

Taylor, C. and White, S. (2000) *Practising Reflexivity in Health and Welfare: Making Knowledge*. Buckingham: Open University Press.

Teater, B. (2010) *An Introduction to Applying Social Work Theories and Methods*. Maidenhead: McGraw Hill/Open University Press.

Thomas, D. (1983) *The Making of Community Work*. London: George Allen & Unwin.

Thompson, N. (1991) *Crisis Intervention Revisited*. Birmingham: PEPAR publications.

Thompson, N. (1993) *Anti-Discriminatory Practice*. Basingstoke: Macmillan.

Thompson, N. (2002) 'Social work with adults', in Adams, R., Dominelli, L. and Payne, M. (eds) *Social Work Themes Issues and Critical Debates*. Basingstoke: Palgrave Macmillan.

Treacher, A. and Carpenter, J. (eds) (1984) *Using Family Therapy*. Oxford: Blackwell.

Trevithick, P. (2005a) *Social Work Skills: a practice handbook*, 2nd edn. Maidenhead: Open University Press.

Trevithick, P. (2005b) 'The knowledge base of groupwork and its importance within social work', *Groupwork*, 15(2), pp. 80–107.

Trotter, C. (2006) *Working with Involuntary Client: a guide to practice*, 2nd edn. London: Sage.

Tsoi, M. and Yule, J. (1982) 'Building up new behaviours: shaping, prompting and fading', in Yule, W. and Carr, J. (eds) *Behaviour Modification for the Mentally Handicapped*. London: Croom Helm.

Tuckman, B. W. and Jensen, M. A. C. (1977) 'Stages of small group development revisited', *Group and Organisation Studies*, 2(4), pp. 419–27.

Tuson, G. (1996) 'Writing postmodern social work', in P. Ford and P. Hayes (eds) *Education for Social Work: Arguments for Optimism*. Aldershot: Avebury (in association with CEDR).

Vanstone, M. (2004) 'A history of the use of groups in probation work: part two – from negotiated treatment to evidence based practice in an accountable service', *Howard Journal of Criminal Justice*, 43(2), 180–222.

Vetere, A. (1999) 'Family therapy', in Hill, M. (ed.) *Effective Ways of Working with Children and their Families*. London: Jessica Kingsley.

Ward, D. (2002) 'Where has all the groupwork gone?', in Adams, R., Dominelli, L. and Payne, M. (eds) *Social Work Themes, Issues and Critical Debates*. Basingstoke: Palgrave Macmillan.

Ward, D. (2009) 'Groupwork', in Adams, R., Dominelli, L. and. Payne, M. (eds) *Critical Practice in Social Work*, 2nd edn. Basingstoke: Palgrave Macmillan.

Waterhouse, L. and McGhee, J. (2002) 'Social work with children and families', in Adams, R., Dominelli, L. and Payne, M. (eds) *Social Work Themes, Issues and Critical Debates*. Basingstoke: Palgrave Macmillan.

Weaver, B. and McNeill, F. (2010) 'Travelling hopefully desistance theory and probation practice', in Brayford, J., Cowe, F. and Deering, J. (eds) *What Else Works? Creative Work with Offenders*. Cullompton: Willan.

Weinberg, A., Williamson, J., Challis, D. and Hughes, J. (2003) 'What do care managers do? A study of working practice in older peoples' services', *British Journal of Social Work*, 33(7), pp. 901–19.

Whitaker, D. S. (1975) 'Some conditions of effective work with groups', *British Journal of Social Work*, 5(4), pp. 423–40.

Whitaker, D. S. (1985) *Using Groups to Help People*. London: Routledge & Kegan Paul.

White, J. (2002) 'Family therapy', in Davies, M. (ed.) *The Blackwell Companion to Social Work*. Oxford: Blackwell.

White, V. (2006) *The State of Feminist Social Work*, London: Routledge.

White, M. and Epston, D. (1990) *Narrative Means to Therapeutic Ends*. New York: Norton.

Wise, S. (1990) 'Becoming a feminist social worker', in Stanley, L. and Wise, S. (eds) *Becoming a Feminist Social Worker*. London: Routledge.

Wittenberg, I. S. (1970) *Psychoanalytic Insight and Relationships: a Kleinian approach*. London: Routledge & Kegan Paul.

Wolfensberger, W. (1983) 'Social role valorisation: a proposed new term for the principle of normalisation', *Mental Retardation*, 21(6), pp. 234–9.

Wootton, B. F. (1959) *Social Science and Social Pathology*. London: George Allen & Unwin.

Yalom, I. D. (1970) *The Theory and Practice of Group Psychotherapy*. New York: Basic Books.

York, A. (1984) 'Towards a conceptual model of community social work', *British Journal of Social Work*, 14, pp. 241–55.

Young, A. M., Ackerman, J. and Kyle, J.G. (2000) 'On creating a workable signing environment: deaf and hearing perspectives', *Journal of Deaf Studies and Deaf Education*, 5(2), pp. 186–95.

Index

abuse
domestic, 34–5, 84, 122
elder, 33, 39
investigating, 69, 76
see also child abuse; domestic
violence
addictive behaviour, 182–4, 188
see also substance abuse
advocacy, 19, 46, 54, 57–61, 93,
112, 218, 268
and children, 211
citizen, 59
for people with learning
disabilities, 59
group, 60
self, 59
types of, 58–60
age, 49, 187
ageism, 53, 119, 122
assessment, 3, 21–44, 48, 67, 69,
72, 76, 93, 107
behavioural, 179–80, 184
communication in, 31
community care, 218, 219,
220, 22
constructivist, 23–4, 115, 123
as CORE, 30–2, 40, 41
exchange model of, 28
of families, 198, 201
framework for, 26, 92
and information technology, 27
models, 29–37
multi-professional, 40–1
narrative assessment, 29, 30, 38
of need, 35–37, 92, 218, 223
observation in, 31

and oppression, 25, 37–9, 41
positivist, 22–3
procedural model, 25–6
questioning model, 24–5
and reflection, 23, 31, 88
and review, 94–5
single shared, 41, 221–2
theories, 22–4
user participation in, 28, 38,
39–40, 54, 157
see also risk assessment
asylum seekers, 82, 138, 198, 261
attachment, 107, 110–11, 114,
119, 130, 154
and grief, 141, 142

Barclay Committee and Report,
262–4
Beck, A.T.,181
behavioural approaches, 129, 161,
239
and assessment, 179–80
critique of, 186–7
techniques of, 180–2
see also cognitive-behaviour
therapy
bereavement, 99, 129, 139–42
assessment in palliative care,
146
dual process model, 141
and loss, 139–40
see also grief
best value, 92, 94

care, 38, 117, 224, 231, 263
as burden, 228